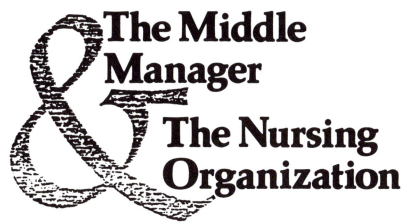

The Middle Manager

& The Nursing Organization

Human Resources
Fiscal Resources

With contributions by:

Ruth R. Alward, R.N., Ed.D.
Assistant Professor
Hunter-Bellevue School of Nursing
Hunter College, City University of New York
New York, New York

Donna M. Costello-Nickitas, R.N., M.S.
Instructor
Hunter-Bellevue School of Nursing
Hunter College, City University of New York
New York, New York

Robert Smith, M.B.A.
Assistant to the Executive Vice President for Nursing
University Hospital
New York University Medical Center
New York, New York

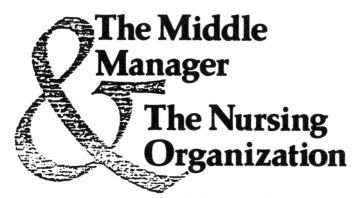

The Middle Manager & The Nursing Organization

Human Resources
Fiscal Resources

Jo Kirsch, R.N., Ed.D.
Director, Graduate Nursing Program
Hunter-Bellevue School of Nursing
Hunter College, City University of New York
New York, New York

APPLETON & LANGE
Norwalk, Connecticut/San Mateo, California

0-8385-6335-X

88 89 90 91 92 / 10 9 8 7 6 5 4 3 2 1

Prentice-Hall of Australia, Pty. Ltd., Sydney
Prentice-Hall Canada, Inc.
Prentice-Hall Hispanoamericana, S.A., Mexico
Prentice-Hall of India Private Limited, New Delhi
Prentice-Hall International (UK) Limited, London
Prentice-Hall of Japan, Inc., Tokyo
Prentice-Hall of Southeast Asia (Pte.) Ltd., Singapore
Whitehall Books Ltd., Wellington, New Zealand
Editora Prentice-Hall do Brasil Ltda., Rio de Janeiro

Library of Congress Cataloging-in-Publication Data

Kirsch, Jo.
  The middle manager and the nursing organization.

  Includes index.
  1. Nursing services—Administration. 2. Nurse
administrators. 3. Middle managers. I. Title.
[DNLM: 1. Financial Management—methods—nurses'
instruction. 2. Nursing staff—organization &
administration. 3. Nursing, Supervisory—methods.
4. Personnel Managment—methods—nurses' instruction.
WY 105 K61m]
RT89.K59 1987   362.1'73'068   87-30749
ISBN 0-8385-6335-X

Production Editor: Carlo R. Francisco
Designer: Steven M. Byrum

362. 173068
K 639 m
1988

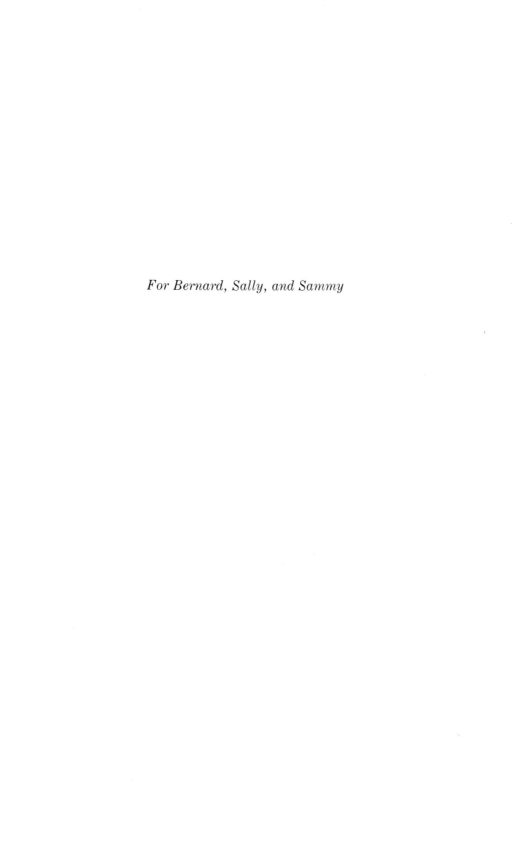

For Bernard, Sally, and Sammy

CONTENTS

PREFACE

This book is written for middle-managers in nursing; both students of nursing management and practicing nurse managers. It addresses the two elements that are essential in a middle manager's work: management of the *human* and *fiscal* resources of the nursing organization. The book departs from most nursing management texts in this two-pronged approach and also in its nontraditional handling of the functions of the manager. The human resources content of the book serves to help develop concepts and expand the manager's thinking about managing people in organizations. The content in fiscal resource management follows a more traditional approach that aims to give the middle manager concrete information and illustrations of management of the nursing budget. It is hoped that having both elements of management in one text will prove useful for the middle manager in nursing.

No book is written without some measure of sacrifice and struggle. I am indebted to those who sacrificed and struggled along with me: contributing authors Ruth Alward, Donna Costello-Nickitas, and Robert Smith; my editor Marion Kalstein-Welch; and most of all my family—Bernard, my husband, friend, and mentor, and my children, Sally and Sammy, who make it all worth it.

INTRODUCTION

The management process has come under close scrutiny in recent years by both management theorists and managers. Although the classical elements of management—planning, organizing, directing, and controlling—are still considered the basic building blocks of good management, some interesting and provocative studies have challenged this commonly held view of managerial work. We now know that up to 80 percent of a manager's time is spent interacting with people. The functions of the manager are not carried out in isolation behind closed doors, but in the give-and-take of personal interactions. Organizations that recognize the crucial importance of the people element of managing have been found to be among the most excellent in the country. Yet, in many nursing organizations whose stated goals are centered on caring, there has been a lack of care shown for the people who provide the caring. One example is the lack of sensitivity to the needs of nurse employees that has been demonstrated over the years in many nursing organizations.

Because an organization's people are its greatest asset, the focus of Human Resources has been chosen for Part I of this book. The elements of planning, organizing, directing, and controlling, used as the basis for many nursing management books, are not used as the basis for this section of the book. Rather, by developing a view of the organization as an open system in which there is congruence between the Task, the People, and the Formal and Informal Organization, a framework for the management of human resources in the nursing organization is presented. Each nurse manager develops a unique style of management, and the theories and concepts presented here serve as a foundation for that style.

Managing the human element of an organization, however important, is of course only half the picture. The management of Fiscal Resources is the other half. This book is unique in that it combines the two most critical nursing management functions into one text. The management of the organization's fiscal resources is of great concern to today's nurse manager. Nurses have traditionally had little or no background in the budget process and in fiscal management until they find themselves in management positions. Some are intimidated by the prospect of managing the budget process; some learn "on the job." Part II of this book will illuminate the budget process and discuss major areas of concern in the fiscal management of the nursing organization in today's climate of financial constraints. Both the experienced and the new middle manager should find useful information for their organizations in the discussion of overall economic trends that affect the nursing organization and the specific elements that make up the nursing organization's budget. Budgeting is presented with detailed examples of one method of calculating the budget for a hospital nursing department. It is recognized that each nursing organization will have some unique budget procedures of its own.

No one book can encompass all of the knowledge and information successful middle managers in nursing will need in their work. This book does not propose to be the ultimate "how to" guide for nursing management. It is proposed as a guide to avenues of thinking and future study and research in these most complex facets of a nurse manager's work — the management of human and fiscal resources. Through the presentation of concepts, models, and philosophies that view the nurse manager's work from both new and traditional perspectives, we hope to guide the nurse manager in managing for excellence.

Part I: Human Resources

The six chapters which encompass the human resource management concepts are organized to present the importance of people and person-to-person interactions in every aspect of the nursing organization's management and the middle manager's work.

Chapter 1 presents a conceptualization of the nursing organization as an open system that requires a close fit between all of the organization's essential elements: input, transformation, and output. Chapter 2 uses Henry Mintzberg's research to present a unique view of managerial work and the nurse manager's roles. Chapter 3 explores models of leadership behavior from the traditional Ohio State Leadership Studies to Burns' view of leadership as transformational rather than transactional. Chapter 4 looks in depth at the most essential element of any nursing organization, the individual. It is individual motivation that holds the key to organizational excellence. Chapter 5 explores the natural groupings that become a part of the nursing organization's informal structure. Groups, political influences, and labor relations and their affects are discussed. Chapter 6 concludes Part I with an exploration of decision-making strategies for the nurse manager. Current theories of decision making by individuals and groups and pitfalls common in the process are discussed.

Part II: Fiscal Resources

Part II of *The Middle Manager and the Nursing Organization: Human Resources—Fiscal Resources* focuses on the complexities involved in the management of the nursing organization's fiscal resources. Major economic influences on nursing's fiscal management are presented, as are specific budgetary concepts with detailed illustrations of areas of innovation for today's nurse manager.

Chapter 7 explores the origin and uses of patient classification systems and their impact on the nursing budget regarding staffing. Chapter 8 presents concepts of basic budgeting that are crucial for developing the nursing budget. Chapters 9 and 10 explore in depth the salary and nonsalary budgets of the nursing organization with detailed illustrations. Chapter 11 concludes Part II with an in depth discussion of the impact of prospective payment systems and marketing concepts for nurse managers.

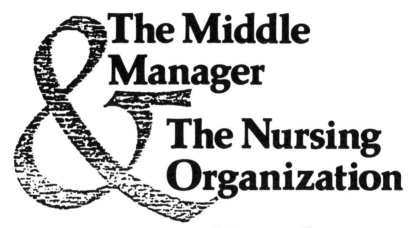

The Middle Manager

Manager

The Nursing Organization

Human Resources
Fiscal Resources

Managing Human Resources

CHAPTER 1

The Nursing Organization as an Open System

Because we experience life as a series of person-to-person contacts, we tend to take organizations for granted and do not notice their existence until a problem or a crisis arises that brings the existence of a particular organization into view. When the employees of a large airline go out on strike leaving thousands of travelers stranded, the airline organization becomes very evident to the public. Patients may describe their hospital stay as one that was satisfactory or not satisfactory depending on the person-to-person contacts made. If the local hospital should be threatened with closure because of financial constraints, however, the patient might then question who in the *organization* is responsible for this turn of events. How then can we define organizations? Simply put, organizations *allow people to accomplish together what individuals could not hope to accomplish alone.*

Most people, when asked to describe an organization, rely on an organizational chart or table of organizations as the basis for their description. But organizations are much more complex than their formal structure alone. Aldrich (1979, p. 4) defines organizations as "goal directed, boundary maintaining, activity systems." Organizations are *goal directed* in that the activities of their members are directed toward a common purpose or task. Organizations *maintain their boundaries* in that they make distinctions between members and nonmembers. "From an organization's perspective, the abilty to maintain boundaries is critical for the maintenance of organizational autonomy" (Aldrich, 1979, p. 5).

Organizations are *activity systems* in that they possess a technology for accomplishing the work of the organization, whether it be processing raw materials or people. Eventually division of labor leads to role differentiation and specialization of functions within the organization. To understand the complexities of the nursing organization and its management, we must first have a grasp of the functioning of the organization as a goal directed, boundary maintaining, activity system.

Open systems theory is helpful in conceptualizing the functions of organizations. Many nurse managers are familiar with open systems theory from their studies of nursing theory and the application of the open systems model to the study of man and health. Open systems theory can help us to describe organizations in general, and the nursing organization and its functioning in particular. Figure 1–1 illustrates the elements that constitute the organization as an open system, namely, *Input, Transformation, Output,* and *Feedback.* Considering the organization as an open system assumes that it is in constant interaction with its environment. Figure 1–1 illustrates the organization as constantly receiving input from the environment. This input is transformed by the processes and functions of the organization into the output or the product. The concept is not complete, however, until we consider the element of strategy, which can be thought of as a catalyst that transforms organizational inputs into output (Nadler, Tushman, and Hatvany, 1982). Feedback about the output (or products) of the organization is constantly fed into the input system and becomes part of the interaction between the organization and the environment.

Each of the elements of the open systems model will be analyzed and defined to understand the nursing organization as an open system.

INPUT

Organizational inputs are those elements that come into the organization from the outside. Included in input are such elements as the environment, the resources, and the history of the organization.

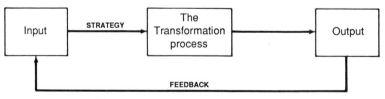

Figure 1–1. A model of an open system.

Environmental Inputs

Environmental inputs include:

- Geographical location of the organization
- Federal, state, and local regulations
- Community needs
- Economic and social climate of the times

There has never been a time when nursing managers have needed to be more knowledgeable about the impact of input elements on their organizations. The 1980s and 1990s will be a time of increasing federal regulation and influence on the financing of health care and health care organizations. Prospective payment plans already have and will continue to have a tremendous impact on fiscal resources and, therefore on the management of the nursing organization. The astute nurse manager realizes that today's legislation about health care will have an impact on the organization tomorrow.

State and local regulations also greatly influence what comes into the organization as a given and will influence decisions such as size, location, and type of services a health care organization delivers. The needs of the community must necessarily affect what the health care organization has as its goal and mission, as does the geographical location of the organization. We must be aware of the influence of demographic changes on delivery of health care. For example, the increase in the number of aged in our population and their health care needs has greatly influenced the direction of health care growth in the last decade. Federal regulations regarding the disbursement of monies for Medicare and Medicaid, whose recipients are primarily the aged, are having a revolutionary effect on budgeting in hospitals throughout the United States. Statewide fiscal restraints have led to changes such as care of the mentally ill outside of large state-financed institutions in some states. The move toward home health care and reimbursement by insurance companies for outpatient as well as inhospital care also affects the directions in which the nursing organization channels its resources. Prospective payment plans will continue to govern the budgets of all hospitals throughout the country and will no doubt force the closure of some of the smaller and perhaps less well-managed hospitals. These are examples of the impact of wider environmental issues on the delivery of health care and nursing services.

Although talk of federal budget deficits may seem far removed from the nurse manager's daily functioning, these issues, seemingly global in scope, will influence the organization daily, whether directly or indirectly.

The environment is a source of information that flows into the organization and directly affects its decision-making. However, an element of uncertainty exists because the effect of information regarding the environment on the functioning of an organization is unpredictable. For example, a nurse manager may be well aware that a prospective payment plan is currently in effect, but may not have a good picture of how this impacts on the nursing organization. Even if able to project possible effects, there is always uncertainty in predicting the influence of environmental elements on the organization with accuracy.

Resource Inputs

Resource inputs include:

- Human resources
- Fiscal resources
- Client resources

The human resources to be considered in the nursing organization include both personnel and clients. In the case of a manufacturing organization, raw materials would be a resource element. In the nursing organization we can consider our client population or pool as an input element, comparable to raw materials for a manufacturing organization. When considering its goal and mission, a health care organization must take into account the community needs that the organization hopes to meet.

What are the *human resources* available to health care organizations in general and the nursing organization in particular? The location of an organization and the type of health care services it delivers, as well as the pool of professional and nonprofessional workers in the community, are of paramount importance in considering the human resources available to the organization. For example, setting up a hospital nursing division with the goal of an all R.N. staff may be unrealistic in a community where the pool of R.N. applicants is low. On the other hand, an acute care hospital in a community with many hospitals, universities, and medical centers would have an excellent pool of R.N. applicants from which to draw.

Adequate *fiscal resource* inputs are fundamental to the operation of any organization. Nursing managers today are increasingly aware of the need to understand the sources of revenue for their organizations and to have control over their allocation. Indeed, mastery of the elements of fiscal resource management is crucial for today's nurse manager. Prospective payment systems will greatly influence the management of the nursing budget in the 1990s. Mastery of fiscal management is so crucial for today's nurse manager that Part II of this text is devoted to the management of fiscal resources in the nursing organization.

History of the Organization

The history of an organization also serves as a source of input. Very few of us have the privilege of beginning with a clean slate by creating new organizations. Most nurse managers find themselves in health care organizations with a history. That history includes the past missions and goals of the organization, the overall development of the organization, key strategic decisions made in the past, as well as the action of past organizational leaders. All of these elements have an impact on the current functioning of the nursing organization. Astute nurse managers learn as much as possible about the history of their organization in the beginning of their tenure. Understanding the history of the nursing organization can give valuable insight into the values, norms, and culture that nurse managers will find within the organization.

STRATEGY

Strategy is the match between organizational resources or input and the organization's missions and goals. An organization's strategy is the element through which its input is transformed into output. It is the *catalyst* that matches the organization's input with the development of its missions and goals. In Figure 1–2, an adaptation of the Nadler–Tushman congruence model is illustrated. The illustration shows that strategy is the element through which input is transformed into output. Strategy implies the concept of choice.

The choices an organization makes about how it will use its input to achieve its goals are the essence of strategic planning.

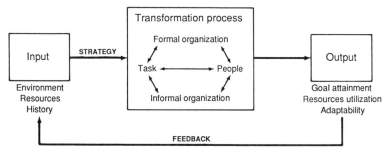

Figure 1–2. An adaptation of the congruence model of organizations. *(After Nadler, Tushman, and Hatvany, 1982.)*

One may define strategy as "the determination of the basic long-run goals and objectives of an enterprise, and the adoption of courses of action and the allocation of resources necessary for carrying out these goals" (Aldrich, 1979, p. 137).

It is in the kinds of strategic choices and plans made by the nursing organization that the concepts of management are wedded to the goals of the nursing organization, thus using the input elements to their best advantage. Stevens points out that "the conceptualization of the care delivery goal varies depending on the nursing theories and philosophies accepted or enacted by a nursing division" (Stevens, 1980, p. VIII). In most nursing organizations today,the goals of the organization are directed toward the care of the patient and the return of that patient to his or her optimum state of health. Traditionally, the goals of the nursing department have been focused on care of patients and delivery of nursing care services. They did not focus on economy, efficiency, or profit motives, as do profit-oriented business, in formulating their strategies. In today's climate of scarce resources, nursing organizations have to formulate goals with cost-effectiveness in mind, as well as basing the structure of the organization on theories and philosophies of nursing synchronous with the goals of the organization.

If strategy is the matching of an organization's resources with its mission and goals, then caution must be used in developing mission and goal statements. The nursing organization must have achievable goals from which strategies can be developed. If the organization is unable to achieve its goals on a regular basis it is demoralizing for the managers and staff alike. If this is the case, the mission and goal statements of the organization should be reconsidered.

OUTPUT

The output of an organization is what it produces. But beyond the basic product produced, one must have a broader view of outputs. The components that contribute to an organization's performance and effectiveness must also be considered part of the output of the system. Examples of the output of a nursing organization follow.

The Products Produced

These would include patient services such as the inpatient, outpatient, and speciality areas that provide nursing care. It might include education of students, staff, and patients, as well as community health education. Also considered a product of a nursing organization would be research in nursing, which contributes to the body of nursing knowledge. The main product of the nursing organization can be considered quality in patient care.

Organizational Performance

How well a nursing organization achieves its goals and meets its objectives is one measure of its performance output. *Resource utilization*, or how well the nursing organization makes use of its available resources is a crucial measure of performance. If the product is produced and the goal met through the resource building rather than resource burning, then the organization is performing effectively.

The functioning of *groups* within the organization is a contributing factor in organizational performance, as is the functioning of individuals. Groups or units at the department, division, or subunit level all contribute to the overall output of the system. At the level of the individual, output is influenced by behavior and reactions such as job satisfaction, stress, and quality of worklife.

Organizational Effectiveness

The components that make an organization effective are complex and have been widely discussed in management literature. Certainly the attainment of goals, the utilization of resources, and the adaptability of the organization are important elements in yielding its effectiveness. Adaptability, or how the nursing organization positions itself in regard to its external and internal environments is crucial to its effectiveness. In other words, is the nursing organization capable of change? To operate as a truly open system, feedback from the environment about performance must be an essential element in future strategic planning for the organization.

THE TRANSFORMATION PROCESS

The *transformation process*, as pictured in Figure 1–2, has as its main elements the *task*, the *formal organization*, the *individual*, and the *informal organization*. The critical element of the Nadler–Tushman model is the *congruence* or "fit" between all of the elements of the transformation process (Nadler, Tushman, and Hatvany, 1982). Let us consider each of these elements individually in terms of the nursing organization. The logical element with which to begin is the *task* of the organization. Task is often said to dictate the structure of an organization, and on close examination, the task of the nursing organization frequently dictates the organizational structure.

Task

The task of the health care organization is related to returning the client to health. It may also have as goals education of medical and nursing personnel, and research, depending on the size and university affiliations of the institution. The task of the nursing organization within a given health care organization is the delivery of nursing care services to the client in an effort to return the client to the optimum level of wellness. It is obvious that the tasks of both the health care organization and the nursing organization require a great deal of professional knowledge and skill in order to be accomplished. The skill of professional nurses, physicians, social workers, laboratory staff, and other health care professionals is essential to the functioning of a well-run health care organization.

There are also needs for ancillary personnel in areas such as general plant maintenance, housekeeping, dietary function, clerical services, and so on. It becomes evident that the task of the nursing organization and the health care organization in general requires many levels of personnel. It requires highly skilled professionals, such as physicians, nurses, and social workers, and the more technical levels of employees, such as laboratory technicians. Semi-skilled labor of nursing assistants and relatively unskilled labor in areas such as housekeeping, dietary, and transportation are also required.

The task of the nursing organization has as a characteristic some degree of uncertainty. Uncertainty is described by organizational theorists as the degree to which the work or the task to be performed by an organization is not routine. Figure 1–3 illustrates the components affecting the tasks of the nursing organization. Certainly there are some elements of routineness in the functions of the nursing organization. However, the constant flow of clients, either in an inpatient or an outpatient facility, the varying kinds of health care problems presented and, in the inpatient facility, the 24-hour nature of the functioning of the nursing organization, all contribute to a degree of uncertainty regarding the nursing organization's task. Therefore, it is difficult to predict what will occur in the future in defining the task of the nursing organization. Although we must make predictions to budget and allocate resources for the day-to-day functioning of the

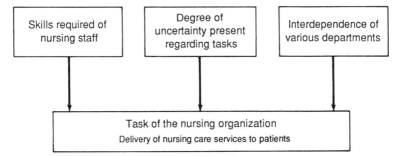

Figure 1–3. Components affecting performance of the task of the nursing organization.

organization, we must also be aware of our inability to predict with total accuracy how the organization's functioning may be altered by changes in the input system.

Also, in times of political uncertainty, when elements in the environment pressure the organization, it may find itself focusing away from its task as defined in the mission and goals statement. If the nursing organization is to develop congruence, its primary task must be clear. To maintain a good fit between the elements of task, individual, and formal and informal structures, the primary task of the organization must be paramount.

The Individual

The individual is perhaps the most crucial element of the transformation process. Without the individual there would be no organization. The element of the individual is so important that Chapter 3 will be devoted to the individual in the nursing organization in detail. Once we have identified the tasks to be performed by the nursing organization and the various levels of skill and knowledge needed to perform these tasks, the characteristics of the individuals to be hired for effective operation of the organization will become apparent. Nurse managers may ask themselves the following questions: What kind of knowledge and skill do the employees in my organization need? What are the individual needs and preferences of the persons that I employ in my organization? What are their expectancies in terms of rewards? What are the intrinsic rewards inherent in the tasks to be performed in the nursing organization? These are the questions to be considered when trying to obtain the best possible fit between the task to be performed and the individual to be selected for the nursing organization (Nadler, Tushman, and Hatvany, 1982).

Our main task in discussing the individual as an element of

the transformation process is to point out the importance of a good match between the tasks to be performed by the organization and the skills of the employees of that organization. The elements of motivation and reward, however, must also match the tasks and the skills of the employees. There must be congruence between, task, skill, motivation, and reward. If, for example, one wished to staff a long-term care facility, the nurse manager would need to employ staff with a different mix of skill levels than would be hired to staff an acute care facility. Determining the level of acuity of patients through patient classification systems helps nurse managers match the numbers of staff and levels of skills of that staff to the nursing tasks to be performed. When the *skills* of the individuals are *well matched* with the *tasks* to be performed, then *congruence* exists between these elements of the transformation process. When equal care is taken to match reward systems to the skills and needs of those individuals who are employed by the organization, the foundation for a motivated, productive staff has been built. If congruence exists between the individual skills, the tasks of the organization, and the rewards offered, then employees are not mere pawns on a chess board, but valued members of a productive team.

The Formal Organization

The formal organization is what most people readily identify as *the* organization when asked to describe their own or another organization. The formal organizational structure is crucial to the functioning and efficiency of the nursing organization. The kinds of structures, processes, and methods through which tasks are performed, and through which individuals learn what is expected of them, are crucial to organizational efficiency. The *design* of the organization, the *structure* of various subunits or departments, the *coordination* between units, and the *control* mechanisms are all elements of importance to the formal organizational design.

The task of the organization helps determine what its structure will be. For example, the kinds of patients a health facility deals with, or the specialties of various physicians and nurses caring for patients, may dictate how patients or clients are grouped together for care in that facility. If a large hospital offers specialty services such as cardiac care, pediatrics, or rehabilitation, those kinds of patients will naturally be grouped together rather than scattered throughout the hospital, both for the patients' well-being, as well as for efficient delivery of care by skilled professionals such as physicians and nurses.

Hospitals, therefore, become divided into subunits or departments with patients of like kind as a natural outgrowth of the tasks to be performed. Certainly it would not be efficient or effective to have patients of very disparate diagnoses together on a unit requiring the care of various professionals with a wide range of skills. If hospitals were not subdivided as they are, one might conceive of ludicrous consequences, such as an obstetrical patient in a room next to a 75-year-old man with a myocardial infarction. The task of caring for patients, therefore, dictates the basic structures of health care organizations, as it does for organizations in general. The design of *jobs* is also an important element of the formal organization. We have frequently *designed* nursing jobs for maximum efficiency in the care of patients, with little regard to the inherent reward in performing tasks for the nursing personnel involved. Job descriptions are *not* job designs. Formal job descriptions are a necessary entity in any organization for employees to understand the basis for evaluation, and for management to understand who has responsibility for various tasks in the organization. The design of jobs, however, is more complex than mere job descriptions. The design of nursing jobs for maximum motivation and efficiency is presented in detail in Chapter 3, The Individual in the Nursing Organization, which discusses the Hackman–Oldham job diagnostic model.

The formal structure of nursing organizations has been evolving for the past several years. *Traditional structures* in many organizations have looked very much like Figure 1–4, which illustrates the traditional hierarchical, many-layered, formal structure that has typified nursing organizations as well as other service and for-profit organizations, for many years. This type of hierarchical structure is described by Mintzberg (1983) as the Machine Bureaucracy. This structure is appropriate in organizations where tasks are simple and repetitive, although not restricted to manufacturing organizations.

> . . . machine bureaucratic work is found, above all, in environments that are simple and stable. The works of complex environments cannot be rationalized into simple tasks, and that of dynamic environments cannot be predicted, made repetitive, and so standardized. (Mintzberg, 1983, p. 171)

Machine bureaucracies are characterized by a *tall* hierarchy of authority in the middle level. These structures may have evolved in nursing organizations when the tasks performed by nurses were of a simpler nature, but have become anachronistic to today's professional nursing environment.

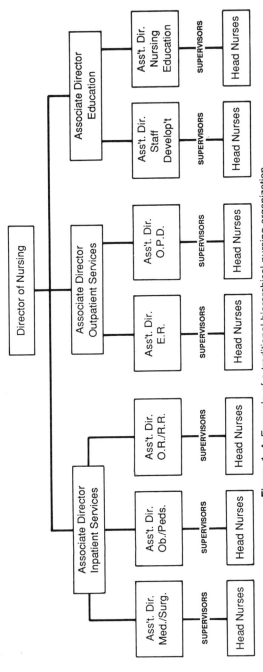

Figure 1–4. Example of a traditional hierarchical nursing organization.

Figure 1–5 shows a nursing organization that has evolved from the traditional hierarchical structure into a more *flattened one*. Notice the absence of the many layers of assistant directors and associate directors of nursing, and the shortened channel of communication between head nurses and the apex of the nursing organization. This structure fits Mintzberg's description of a professional bureaucracy. The professional bureaucracy "hires duly trained and indoctrinated specialists—professionals—for the operating core, and gives them considerable control over their own work" (Mintzberg, 1983, p. 190). It is different from the machine bureaucracy in the flatness of its middle level and is, therefore, a more decentralized structure. The professional bureaucracy is still a bureaucratic organization; however, the work standards of the organization are generated outside of the organization's structure.

> . . . the standards of the Professional Bureaucracy originates largely outside its own structure, in self governing associations its operators join with their colleagues from the Professional Bureaucracies. These associations set universal standards, which they make sure are taught by the universities and used by all the bureaucracies of the profession. (Mintzberg, 1983, p. 192)

The sources of authority are less hierarchical in nature than in the traditional structure of a machine bureaucracy. The authority and power in professional bureaucracies arises from professional expertise. The move to a more flattened structure is probably the most beneficial change in structure for most nursing organizations. A professional bureaucratic structure increases autonomy and responsibility for those at the operating level of the organization—a need felt by many of today's professional nurses. Whatever the formal structure under which the nursing organization operates, it must allow for the high degree of *interdependence* with other members of the health care team.

The Informal Organization

The informal organization is the element that has been least identified by nurse managers in traditional descriptions of organizational functioning. The importance of the informal organization is being recognized in current management literature. The informal organization takes into consideration: *leadership behavior, intergroup* and *intragroup relations*, informal *working relationships* above and beyond the formal structure of the organization, and the various kinds of *communication patterns* and *networking* with the organization. The informal organization is the *invisible*

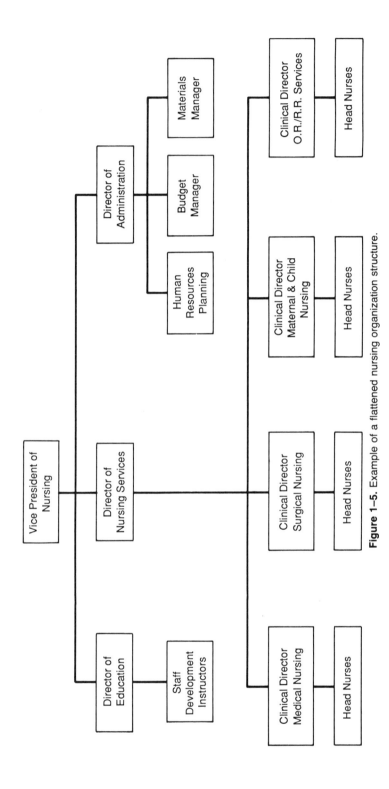

Figure 1–5. Example of a flattened nursing organization structure.

organization. Although we can list the individuals in the organization, define their tasks, and chart the formal channels of communication, it is the informal organization that is more difficult to identify, and to use to our best advantage. We can identify on an organizational chart who the leader of a group or an organizational subunit is *supposed* to be. However, we cannot always identify who our informal leaders are. Who are the leaders chosen by peers because of expertise or charismatic leadership ability?

Knowing who the natural leaders of a group are may assist managers greatly in implementing change within an organization. Using those informal leaders respected by their peers, to work with them on change, is an example of how nurse managers can effectively tap into the informal organization.

Relationships within groups and between groups can be a source of either constructive movement for an organization, or of destructive holding back of progress. If there is intragroup conflict or intergroup conflict, it can slow down the efficiency of the organization. How can the nurse manager use the politics, networking, and coalitions of the organization to the best advantage? Chapter 4, The Group and the Nursing Organization, will consider in depth those areas that are crucial to the understanding of networking and politics within the nursing organization. All of us use the informal organization every day. Think about how we may pick up the phone and call a friend in another department for information we would like to have that may be weeks in forthcoming through the normal organizational channels. A nurse manager who believes that the staff is ignorant of some changes that are being planned, may be surprised to find that through the "grapevine" they have gotten wind of this long before the planned announcement. It becomes evident that for effective functioning of the organization, the nurse manager must understand these forceful informal elements and how to use them.

Another important factor to consider when discussing the informal organization is *organizational culture.* Management theorists are becoming more and more aware of the importance of the culture of an organization to its functioning. What is organizational culture? The culture of an organization is a combination of its *norms, values,* and *roles.* "A particular organization will share certain norms with others of its type and some norms with organizations in general, but it will also have its own taboos, folk ways, and mores" (Katz and Kahn, 1978, p. 50).

Although a hospital may have certain functions in common with a university, or even a factory, these organizations all have their unique norms, values, and roles. Even hospitals and other health care facilities, although sharing some common norms and values, will differ greatly in climate or culture from one organization to another. The values of an organization are set out in some part by its philosophy, goal, and mission statement. However, how these values are reinterpreted by the informal organization greatly influences the organization's culture or climate. Although members of a particular organization may not always be able to furnish concrete information about the culture of their organization, an astute manager can observe those elements that are unique to a particular organization. Much in the same way an anthropologist becomes a *participant observer* in a culture, a nurse manager can become a participant observer in the organization.

The elements that make up an organization's culture are: its *history*, which includes its origins and struggles, both internal and external; the *kinds of people* the organization attracts; and elements such as its *physical facilities* and *layout*.

Facilities offered by an organization, for both clients and staff, can tell us a great deal about what the organization values. Are working conditions pleasant for staff? Where is the staff cafeteria? Are client facilities clean, pleasant, and safe? Answers to questions such as these will be revealing of what an organization values.

Behavior of employees gives us an idea of the norms of an organization. Are employees expected to adhere to a particular dress code? Is it rigid? Is it relaxed? Are there comfortable facilities provided for employees? How are visitors to the organization received? All of these small observations added together can give one a sense of a particular organization's culture. If managers hope to make changes and have growth in the organization, it behooves them to understand the culture of the organization. Determining what the norms of the organization are, what it values, and bringing these norms and values to the surface in feedback sessions is one helpful way of beginning change. Indeed, Katz and Kahn have defined organizational integration as "a fusion of role, norm and value components" (1978, p. 44).

Roles are sets of behaviors that are defined by the organization. Usually they can be found in job descriptions. People behave in organizational roles in ways that are determined by their own personalities, their understanding of what is expected of them by others, and their desire to conform to the norms and values of the organization. If roles are unclear there may be conflict and ambiguity. In an organization where roles are clearly defined, and the values of the organization truly reflect their mission and goals, the nurse manager will find the devel-

TABLE 1–1. FIT NEEDED AND ISSUES RAISED IN CONGRUENCE MODEL OF ORGANIZATIONS

Fit Needed	Issues Raised
Individual—Formal Organization	Do individuals understand the organization's structure? Does organization structure provide for meeting needs of individuals? Are organization goals and individual goals congruent?
Individual—Task	Does the staff have the skills and abilities needed to perform tasks? Is the work of the organization designed to meet individual needs?
Individual—Informal Organization	Does the informal organization meet individual needs? Does the informal organization use individual resources?
Task—Formal Organization	Does the organization structure facilitate the demands of the task? Does the organization structure provide motivation to meet the task?
Task—Informal Organization	Does the informal organization structure facilitate task performance? Does the informal structure hinder meeting the task demands?
Formal Organization—Informal Organization	Is the culture of the informal organization consistent with the structures, goals, and reward systems of the formal organization?

opment of norms that support integration within the nursing organization.

The fit or congruence between the four elements of the transformation process has been demonstrated to be of crucial importance. We cannot consider each of these elements individually, but must look at the interconnection, or fit, between task, individual, informal organization, and formal organization. Table 1–1 illustrates the fits necessary between the elements of the transformation process and highlights those issues that are raised in working toward a good fit between these elements of the organization (Nadler, Tushman, and Hatvany, 1982, p. 43).

REFERENCES AND BIBLIOGRAPHY

Aldrich, H. *Organizations and environments*. Englewood Cliffs, N.J.: Prentice Hall, 1979.

Davis, T., & Lawrence, P. *Matrix*. Reading, Mass.: Addison-Wesley, 1977.

Galbaith, J.R. *Organization design*. Reading, Mass.: Addison-Wesley, 1977.

Katz, D., & Kahn, R.L. *The social psychology of organizations* (2nd ed.). New York: Wiley, 1978.

Kimberly, J., & Miles, R. *The organizational life cycle*. San Francisco: Jossey-Bass, 1980.

March, J., & Simon, H. *Organizations*. New York: Wiley, 1958.

Mintzberg, H. *Structure in fives: Designing effective organizations*. Englewood Cliffs, N.J.: Prentice Hall, 1983.

Nadler, D., Tushman, M., & Hatvany, N. *Managing organizations: Readings and cases*. Boston: Little, Brown, 1982.

Schein, E. *Organizational culture and leadership*. San Francisco: Jossey-Bass, 1985.

Stevens, B. *The nurse as executive* (2nd ed.). Wakefield, Mass.: Nursing Resources Inc., 1980.

Weber, M. *[The theory of social and economic organization.]* (A. M. Henderson & T. Parsons, trans.) New York: Oxford University Press, 1947.

Weick, K.E. *The social psychology of organizing*. Reading, Mass.: Addison-Wesley, 1969.

CHAPTER 2

The Middle Manager in the Nursing Organization

To discuss the management of the nursing organization's human and fiscal resources, we must first understand what it is that a nurse manager actually does. Many nursing management texts have followed the traditional management concepts of POSDCARB. Nurse managers plan, organize, staff, direct, coordinate, report, and budget, according to this traditional view of the manager's work. Each of these classical elements of management are important and cannot be overlooked. Strategic planning, planning and organizing facilities, information systems, and marketing fall under the planning, organizing, and controlling functions of the POSDCARB model and are of great importance to the success of the nursing organization. However, the notion of the middle manager systemically following these classical management steps in the daily organizational routine is not quite accurate. Indeed, nurse managers might question their managerial efficacy if they measured themselves only against the classical management elements. We know now that 80 percent or more of a manager's time is spent interacting with others, and although they do plan, organize, direct, and control, they do it mostly through personal interaction. The work of Henry Mintzberg puts into perspective the managers' work vis-à-vis interaction with others, which accurately reflects the role of the nurse manager.

In 1973, Mintzberg challenged the POSDCARB approach to the definition, classification, and teaching about management and managerial work. Mintzberg's pioneering research into the nature of managerial work put the concept of management in a new perspective. To fully understand the management role, it is crucial for a successful nurse manager to go beyond the classical POSDCARB conceptualization of management. In Mintzberg's work we find a fresh perspective and a more realistic view of what a nurse manager may actually be called upon to do in that role. Mintzberg's research with top managers led him to propose a set of ten working roles of the manager. These roles are conceptualized in three major categories: *interpersonal, informational,* and *decisional* roles.

THE INTERPERSONAL MANAGEMENT ROLES

The interpersonal management roles described by Mintzberg are those of *figurehead, leader,* and *liaison.* These roles derive from the manager's authority and status in the organization.

Figurehead

The role of *figurehead* is the simplest of all managerial roles. Because of the position of managers in the organization, they are required to perform various symbolic, legal, inspirational, or ceremonial duties. There are times when no one but the director of nursing will do at various important committee meetings throughout a hospital organization. Indeed, it is believed that the figurehead role is most important at the highest levels of the organization. The throwing out of the first baseball of the season by the President of the United States is an example of the role of figurehead in sports in America.

Leader

The second of the interpersonal roles is the role of *leader.* The leader role describes and defines the interpersonal relationships of the manager with his or her subordinates. This is the role that has been given most attention in the management literature. It is the most widely recognized of all managerial roles. In the role of leader, the manager must attempt to motivate subordinates, take responsibility for hiring, training, promotion, and firing of subordinates, and in general create a milieu in the organization that allows for effective achievement of organizational goals.

The leadership role is important enough to warrant closer examination and Chapter 5 is devoted to the concepts of leadership in the nursing organization.

Liaison

The third interpersonal role that the manager carries out is the *liaison* role. This role focuses on the manager's dealings with people outside of his or her own organization. This role may be thought of as a boundary-spanning role. In other words, the manager acts as the go-between for the organization and the outside environment. This liaison function may also include the immediate external environment of the subunit. The higher up on the organizational ladder, the more called upon a manager will be to perform the liaison role. In the role of liaison, the manager develops a network of contacts that can be used to obtain information that may be useful for future negotiations. The chief executive officer has a larger liaison role outside of the organization than does a middle manager. The middle manager in nursing may find the liaison role to be more internal. The liaison serves as a go-between in communications, good relationships, and networking within the subunit of the nursing organization and the health care organization as a whole. The roles of leader and liaison actually confer upon the manager a great deal of privileged information and access to every subordinate in the organization. Enactment of the role provides the nurse with a great deal of current, up-to-date information that can be used to the manager's advantage in decision making.

THE INFORMATIONAL ROLES

The informational roles are those of *monitor, disseminator,* and *spokesman.*

Monitor

As a *monitor,* the manager is constantly seeking and receiving internal and external information from many sources to obtain a thorough knowledge of the environment and the organization. Much of the information received in the monitor role is of an informal nature and is received primarily through verbal contacts, written reports, and observational tours of the organization. A manager who does not make contact with subordinates by touring the organization and speaking with them may have a poorly developed monitor function. To avoid this, it is recommended that new managers spend most of their time in the monitor and liaison roles to build up their information base about the organization. The old cliché that "no news is good news" is not an accurate one for the nurse manager to follow. The nurse manager must perform the monitoring role if he or she is to have accurate data about what is occurring within the organization and be able to spot trouble before it develops.

Disseminator

As a *disseminator*, the role of the manager is to transmit information received from outsiders into the organization. As a disseminator of information, the nurse manager allows subordinates access to some of the privileged information that is available only to him or her. Some of this information may be factual and some of it may be in the form of values about the organization and the forces that influence it. The disseminator role allows the nurse manager to share some of the "power," in the form of crucial information, with subordinates.

Spokesman

The *spokesman* role is the reverse side of the disseminator role. The spokesman transmits information about the organization to outsiders. This may mean people outside the immediate organizational unit, or to the wider organization or environment in general. The manager as spokesman is a public relations person for the organization. The spokesman role is crucial for the nurse manager in defining the organization to outsiders. The way that a nurse manager's unit or subunit is viewed by others within the organization and outside of the organization is due in part to how well he or she plays the spokesman role. The informational roles, then, are crucial to the health and well-being of the nursing organization. If, indeed, information is power, the importance of the nurse manager as a monitor of information and a spokesman about the organization cannot be minimized.

THE DECISIONAL ROLES

The decisional roles are those of *entrepreneur, disturbance handler, resource allocator*, and *negotiator*.

Entrepreneur

In the role of *entrepreneur* the nurse manager will be responsible for initiating change. Mintzberg envisions the entrepreneurial role of the manager as one in which he or she continually searches for opportunities to solve problems and to initiate improvement through change in the organization. Managers may initiate several projects and have them in various stages of development under their more or less direct supervision at one time.

The strategy of the organization is made through the four decisional roles. The degree to which the nurse manager takes an entrepreneurial interest in the organization is the degree to which change and improvement will occur in that organization.

Disturbance Handler

The more a nurse manager is involved in the day-to-day work of the organization, the more likely he or she is to be heavily involved in the role of *disturbance handler*. Disturbances are inevitable in any organization. They can arise in organizations because of insensitivity, but they can also arise in organizations where innovation is intense. When situations arise with which no one is familiar, the nurse manager becomes the organization's "generalist" and disturbance handler, guiding the organization through difficult times. The role of disturbance handler can also include problems of conflict resolution, which is covered in Chapter 4.

Resource Allocator

It is through the role of *resource allocator* that the nurse manager maintains control of the strategy of the organization. Nurse managers have for a long time managed certain human resource aspects of the organization, i.e., maintaining control of the scheduling and assignment of staff. The allocation of fiscal resources is a new role to many middle managers in nursing. Mintzberg has defined three major functions for the resource allocator. The first is the scheduling of the manager's own time. How nurse managers decide to use their time will indicate to the staff those tasks and accomplishments that are valued. This can impact greatly on the formation of the organization's culture.

Second, nurse managers design the basic work of the unit or subunit. The director of nursing, as the chief executive officer of the nursing organization, represents the level of management from which the design of work for the nursing staff comes. However, work design may come from lower levels of management as well. In many hospitals, the drive for primary nursing has begun with staff themselves and the change has been a "bottoms-up" change. Third, managers maintain ultimate control by authorizing major decisions that are made in the organization. For example, if primary nursing is instituted in an inpatient facility, the cost of this change in the delivery of nursing services must be justified by nurse managers in the budget. They must take responsibility for authorizing the change. The resource allocator role is one of the most complex with which managers deal. Frequently the issues are complex, and the time to make decisions is short. Nurse managers must use all the tools at their disposal, basing the decisions on models and conceptual frameworks congruent with their view of the organization.

Negotiator

The final decisional role is that of *negotiator*. The negotiator role is one in which the manager deals with those outside of the organization, in contrast with the disturbance handler role, which focuses on problems within the organization. Examples of the role of negotiator would be the part played by the nurse manager in labor contract negotiations for the staff, or in justifying the budget to superiors in the organization.

It can be seen from Mintzberg's (1973) description of the ten managerial roles that managers do much more than plan, organize, staff, control, direct, and budget in their organization. They maintain a number of more complex and interesting roles that are often performed simultaneously. Mintzberg's research showed that a manager's activities are "characterized by brevity, variety, and fragmentation" (p. 171). In his studies he found that managers show signs of preference for brevity and interruption of their work. They choose activities where they can be current, and where they are in nonroutine situations.

> The manager's work is essentially that of communication and his tools are the five basic media—mail, telephone, unscheduled meetings, scheduled meetings, and tours. (Mintzberg, 1973, p. 171)

Managers clearly favor the verbal media, spending up to 80 percent of their time in verbal communication. To view the nurse manager as one who is removed from staff, deliberating reports, is inaccurate. As many nurse managers already know, they spend a good deal of their time—like the managers in Mintzberg's study—in verbal communication. "Managers in the service organizations spend more time in the liaison role than those in private industry" (p. 97).

This statement demonstrates that the liaison role, again a verbal contact role, is an extremely important one for nurse managers. As we move down the organizational hierarchy, managers at lower levels spend more time in the roles of disturbance handler and negotiator. These managers are more concerned with the steady flow of work and the direct supervision of staff than managers at higher levels. Mintzberg also points out that as organizations become more complex, managers begin to deal with more complex coalitions within the organization. Therefore, the manager will spend more and more time in the roles of *figurehead, liaison, spokesman,* and *negotiator.*

Table 2–1 identifies how the nurse manager functions in each of Mintzberg's managerial roles. The distinction between the functions of the executive level and the middle level manager are illustrated in the examples given.

MANAGERIAL JOB TYPES

In contrast to the dichotomous notion of either an autocratic or a democratic type of manager, Mintzberg has identified *eight managerial job types* that managers fall into. A manager will function as a given "type" depending on the *situation* and *personal characteristics* of the manager. Table 2–2 illustrates the managerial job types and the key management roles to which they correspond. Because the types are linked to situations and personality, managers may function as different types at different times, and in more than one type simultaneously.

Contact Man

The first managerial job type described is that of *contact man.* The contact person is one who spends a great deal of time outside of the organization in the roles of *liaison* and *figurehead.* In service organizations in particular, chief executive officers may fall into this category. Many deans and directors of nursing spend a great deal of time outside of the organizations to develop the reputation of their organizations. Delivering papers, attending workshops, delivering workshops, being present at important professional and organizational meetings in the role of figurehead, all enhance the nursing organization in the eyes of the nursing community and the community at large.

Political Manager

The *political manager* is characterized by the *spokesman* and *negotiator* roles. Many managers in service organizations, such as hospitals, find themselves acting as negotiators or spokesmen for the organization. The political manager spends much of the time dealing with people outside of the organization. In the nurs-

TABLE 2–1. FUNCTIONS OF THE NURSE MANAGER (EXECUTIVE AND MIDDLE LEVEL) IN MINTZBERG'S MANAGERIAL ROLES

	Interpersonal Roles		
	Figurehead	*Leader*	*Liaison*
Executive Level	Represents the nursing organization with appropriate committees and boards, inside and outside of the organization.	Defines the philosophy and goals of the nursing organization. Formulates policy procedure and structure of the nursing organization. Has responsibilities for hiring and firing middle level managers and support staff.	Serves as liaison for the nursing organization with professional and community groups. Relates to governmental and regulatory groups as representative of the nursing organization.
Middle Level	Represents the subunit (department, division) at organizational meetings and committees.	Implements philosophy and goals of the nursing organization. Directs and supervises delivery of services at the subunit level. Has responsibilities for hiring, training, and firing subordinates.	Serves as a liaison for the subunit with other professional groups in the organization. Serves as a member/officer of professional and community groups.

	Informational Roles		
	Monitor	*Disseminator*	*Spokesman*
Executive Level	Establishes and manages information and reporting systems for the organization. Receives input about the organization from internal monitoring. Assesses the impact of external influences on the organization. Monitors the use of resources.	Designs formal communications systems. Provides members with valuable information from inside and outside the organization. Communicates regularly with middle level managers.	Speaks for the nursing organization at meetings and conferences inside and outside of the organization. Defines the organization for outsiders. Represents the nursing organization to V.I.P. visitors.

Middle Level	Implements reporting systems and information systems at the subunit level. Receives reports, makes rounds, and is visible and available to staff. Monitors quality of care, use of personnel, equipment, and supplies at subunit level.	Communicates organization policy to subordinates. Provides subordinates with feedbacks regarding information of importance. Holds regular conferences and meetings and is available to staff for communication.	Speaks for the subunit at meetings and conferences with nursing executives and with other health care professionals. Represents the nursing organization to physicians, family, and visitors.

Decisional Roles

	Entrepreneur	Disturbance Handler	Resource Allocator	Negotiator
Executive Level	Determines strategy and plans for the nursing organization. Initiates change and improvement in delivery of nursing services.	Manages and guides the organization in times of change and unrest. Handles disturbances on an organization-wide level.	Determines and organizes the services, positions, and functions of the nursing organization. Provides resources and determines budget for personnel, equipment, supplies, and education. Schedules and manages own time.	Negotiates with other major services and departments in the health care organization. Negotiates labor contracts.
Middle Level	Participates in strategy formation. Seeks ways to initiate and implement change in the delivery of nursing services.	Manages and guides the subunit in times of change and unrest. Handles disturbances at the subunit level.	Determines budget for subunit and distributes resources to meet the needs of the subunit. Provides for economical use of resources. Schedules and manages own time.	Negotiates with other subunits and executive levels for resources. Participates in labor contract negotiation.

TABLE 2–2. MINTZBERG'S EIGHT MANAGERIAL JOB TYPES

Managerial Job Type	Key Roles
Contact Man	Liaison, Figurehead
Political Manager	Spokesman, Negotiator
Entrepreneur	Entrepreneur, Negotiator
Insider	Resource Allocator
Real-Time Manager	Disturbance Handler
Team Manager	Monitor, Spokesman
New Manager	Liaison, Monitor

ing organization, with so many political pressures from above and below, nurse managers may often find themselves cast in the role of political managers. Thus, they may find themselves spending a good part of the time in meetings with those above them in the hierarchy and in explaining the actions of the organization to special interest groups and coalitions within the organization.

Entrepreneur

The third managerial type is the *entrepreneur*. Most of the entrepreneurial manager's time is spent looking for opportunities to initiate or implement change within the organization. To quote Mintzberg, "The entrepreneur is commonly found at the head of a small, young business organization, where innovation is the key to survival" (p. 128). Mintzberg believes that entrepreneurs are short-lived in large organizations where change and innovations can only be tolerated for short periods of time. So we might look for the entrepreneurial nurse manager in the new facility, or a newly appointed subdivision of a larger facility that is undergoing change. This kind of manager likes change and likes to implement it. He or she might have difficulties in large organizations that are resistant to change.

Insider

The *insider* type is mainly concerned with the smooth running of the organization. These managers have spent time building up the structure of the organization, developing and training their subordinates, and overseeing the operations of the organization in general. The chief roles of the insider are those of *resource allocator* and *leader*. Most middle managers fall into the category of insider managerial type, their main goal being to build up and maintain a stable organization. Frequently, the second person in command assumes the insider role because the chief executive officer is performing in the role of contact person or political manager.

Real-Time Manager

The *real-time manager* is one whose primary role is that of *disturbance handler*. This type of manager is concerned with the maintenance of the internal operations of the organization. However, the focus is primarily on the day-to-day work of the organization and insuring that it continues without interruption. The real-time manager's work is typical of what has been described by Mintzberg as highly fragmented: brief contacts with little time to read mail or give reports. The real-time manager is prepared for all eventualities; has a finger in every pie. In nursing, many head nurses could be characterized as real-time managers. They may be prepared to substitute for an employee, doing the job themselves if necessary, and are found in the basic line positions of head nurse or assistant head nurse in the nursing organization.

Real-time managers are found in organizations that are dynamic, competitive, or high-pressure environments. This certainly characterizes the nursing organization.

Team Manager

The *team manager* is also concerned with an orientation to the internal organization rather than the external environment. However, as differentiated from the insider-type manager and the real-time manager, the team manager is basically concerned with the creation of a team that will perform as a cohesive group and function effectively as a whole. This type of manager excels when the organizational task is difficult to coordinate and yet requires coordination among groups of highly skilled experts. Many nurse managers coordinate the skills of experts in their organizations and may fall into the team manager category, especially those in nursing units where many other professionals are required to maintain effective patient care. For example, intensive care units, or specialized operating room areas require this effort. A team manager is primarily concerned with the *leader role*. The nurse who operates as a team manager must have a great deal of leadership skill and ability.

Expert Manager

The *expert manager* is described as having the key roles of *monitor* and *spokesman*. This type of manager is usually the head of a specialist staff group and serves chiefly as the disseminator and gatherer of information who is consulted about special problems.

In the nursing organization, the *clinical specialist* may function in the role of expert manager. Much of the work is associated with the specialty function, and the clinical specialist functions with fewer of the characteristics of managerial work described for the real-time manager: fragmentation, brevity, and variety. Expert managers have more time to read and write and tend to encounter less pressure and less fragmentation in their work. The value of the expert nurse manager can readily be seen as the head of a group that serves as a nerve center for specialized information in a nursing organization where other nurse managers are involved as entrepreneurs, real-time managers, contact persons, or political managers. The value of the clinical specialist as expert manager can help clarify a role that can at times be ambiguous.

New Manager

The last managerial type is the *new manager*. This manager is obviously new to the job. The newness of the position causes a concentration on the roles of *liaison* and *monitor* as the new manager attempts to build up a web of contacts, or a network and a data base of information from which to function. New managers do not function in the decisional roles for some time; not until they have enough information with which to operate. Mintzberg points out that after new managers have information, they are likely to operate as entrepreneurs and will stay in the entrepreneurial role for some time. Perhaps it is natural for new managers to want to implement change and put their distinctive stamp on the organization. Eventually, new managers will settle into one of the other managerial roles, depending on the needs of the situation and the personal characteristics of the individual in the situation. Because nurse managers work in service organizations, they are more likely to find themselves in the liaison role than would a manager in private industry. The liaison role is characterized by the managerial types, *contact man* and *new manager*, which have been described. Mintzberg states:

> Top Managers of public organizations and institutions spend more time in formal activity such as scheduled clocked meetings and more time meeting directors and outside groups than do managers of private organizations. (1973, p. 130)

Managers at lower levels are oriented more directly toward maintaining a steady work flow than those at higher levels; hence the former spend more time in the real-time roles of disturbance handler and negotiator. The lower the level, the more pronounced are the characteristics of brevity and fragmentation. The focus on current and specific issues is also greater at lower levels of management.

Mintzberg's delineation of the ten managerial roles and the characterization of eight managerial types have impact and value for our analysis of the nurse manager's work. His research did not end with descriptions of what managers do, but went on to give points for more effective managing, which are invaluable for the nurse manager.

TEN POINTS FOR MORE EFFECTIVE MANAGING

1. *Sharing information.* Nurse managers are exposed to a great deal of privileged information and must decide which information will be shared with subordinates and how to disseminate this information. Only those subordinates who are closest to the nurse manager will be privy to much of the information that the nurse manager receives. Therefore, the nurse managers must make conscious decisions about dissemination of information to various units of the organization. Subordinates depend on nurse managers for the information on which they will base their decision making. They also rely on nurse managers to specify what the organizational goals are, and look to nurse managers for a sense of direction and a plan. Because most of the information that nurse managers receive may be verbal in nature, nurse managers must make a conscious effort to document that information and disseminate it efficiently. Even those people who are in convenient verbal reach should receive things in writing occasionally. Managers must decide the confidentiality of information to be documented. Information is a source of power; therefore, nurse managers may fear that giving out information dissipates their power base. However, managers who hoard information may be trading off effectiveness for power. Mintzberg points out that there is more value in having well-informed subordinates who can make effective decisions than in hoarding information as a source of power.
2. *Dealing consciously with superficiality.* Because superficiality is an occupational hazard of nurse managers whose work is characterized by variety, fragmentation, and brevity, they must make a conscious effort to deal with

the tendency toward superficiality. It is easy to continuously operate on a superficial level so that nothing is
dealt with in much depth or detail; it is a hazard that
nurse managers must guard against. Nurse managers
must guard against superficiality by finding a balance
between those issues that require some depth of understanding and judgment on their part, and those that do
not. A great number of issues can be delegated to subordinates who have time to deal with them in more detail
than nurse managers do. There are also those issues that
nurse managers must deal with in some way, but not
necessarily in depth. They can be handled in a more
marginal way. When managers do this, however, they
must realize that they understand these issues only su-
perficially, and that despite their general knowledge,
they might know less than some of the subordinates about
specific details of those issues they do not deal with in
depth. The issues that require the special attention of
managers are the most important and complex ones that
come across the desk. These may be the most sensitive
ones and frequently relate to reorganizing the structure
of the organization, expanding the organization, or dealing with major conflicts within the organization. Even
these most complex issues, which require the manager's
attention in depth, will be dealt with only intermittently
over a period of time. Managers rarely have time to
become so involved with an issue that they can work on
it over a long period, neglecting other duties, unless it
is an organizational emergency.

3. *Sharing the job if information can be shared.* Mintzberg
recommends that one way to overcome a very heavy
managerial workload, particularly at the top levels of an
organization, is to create a management team, or a chief
executive, in which two or three people share a single
job. The problem with sharing the managerial role is
that certain roles cannot be divided; for example, the
monitor role must be held by each member of the management team because they must have full information.
They cannot behave as spokesmen, liaisons, or negotiators unless they have full information. The main disadvantage of sharing a managerial job is the time consumed in simply transmitting information from one
member of the management team to another. Job sharing
at the top managerial ranks is a difficult thing to accomplish. However, it may be worthy of careful considera-

tion in situations where the chief executive officer's position is extremely demanding. Many large nursing organizations today have vice presidents as chief executive officers of the nursing department who work with a management team consisting of a director of nursing and other directors who are directly involved with the in-house operation of the organization. The complexity of the managerial role in these large organizations has been recognized and the chief executive officer serves in the role of monitor, spokesman, liaison, and at times negotiator whereas the directors may serve in the roles of political manager, entrepreneur, and insider.

4. *Making the most of obligations*. Because of the position nurse managers hold, there will be many demands on their time in terms of the obligations they must meet. Successful managers can turn those obligations to their own advantages. What is an obligation to one manager becomes an opportunity to another. The wise manager can see in every obligatory situation an opportunity to accomplish his or her own purposes. Indeed, the transformational leader envisioned by Burns is one who sees no opportunity as too insignificant to articulate his or her values or visions for the organization. While performing the role of figurehead for an organization, the nurse manager may have a chance to gain valued information. A word of caution about making the most of obligation is necessary. Many of the obligations that nurse managers find themselves with are of their own creation. Frequently, early in a new managerial job, nurse managers may set up liaisons, contacts, and information channels by joining organizations and professional groups that later require attention and effort. Perhaps some of these early commitments are made without the full realization of the eventual demands on the manager's time. A wise manager, then, in the early days of tenure, will carefully select only those commitments he or she wants to make and foresees as having value for the future of the organization.

5. *Freeing oneself from obligations*. Nurse managers must make their own free time. It is not easily found in the manager's job. Nurse managers must force free time into their schedule. However, just leaving blank spaces in a diary will not do, as these blank spaces tend to get filled up by callers, people dropping in, last minute meetings, and so on. The great blank space of time for planning

that managers have left in the diary disappears rapidly. If nurse managers have things that *they* specifically want to do, they should schedule them. If there is a project they want to initiate, they should initiate it and require reports of people about the project. If they wish to keep in close touch with what is actually happening to the unit, they should pencil in the time needed to tour the facility. They must commit themselves to it, so that others expect and are waiting for them. If a commitment of this kind is made, time will not get eaten up by other obligations. "Between the mail, the callers, and the crises; not to mention the ever hovering subordinate waiting for a free moment, the passive manager will find no free time to address the major, but not pressing issues" (Mintzberg, p. 181).

6. *Emphasizing the role that fits the situation.* Although the nurse manager should be able to perform all of the basic managerial roles outlined by Mintzberg, most managers will give special attention to certain roles in certain situations. For instance, in governmental organizations and service organizations managers may have to spend extra time in the liaison or spokesman role. Depending on what is happening in an organization, a manager may have to concentrate on the disturbance handler role for a time. The choice of which role to emphasize must reflect what is happening in the organization. Mintzberg's study suggests certain patterns in the roles that managers take on. In a new job, a manager who lacks information will devote considerable time to developing liaisons and to building information channels. When he or she feels more secure about knowledge of the organization, he or she may gradually shift into the role of entrepreneur. After the manager has initiated considerable change in the entrepreneurial role for a period, the manager may find that the organization needs to regain its stability and may return to an emphasis on the leader and disturbance handler role. The key is that the manager must be aware of the role that suits the situation.

7. *Seeing a comprehensive picture in terms of its detail.* Although nurse managers are always working with small pieces of the organization at any one time, they must never lose sight of the whole picture. Nurse managers deal with raw data that they must sift through to have a broad overall picture and model of what is happening in the organization. They must not lose sight of the great

influence that the managerial position offers in an organization. Whether it is a large or a small organization, it is important to remember the great degree of influence that a manager has. Seeing the broad picture in terms of its details requires that managers have a conceptualization about organizations, and a management model by which they function. Nurse managers also must have a theory or model of nursing on which they base the decisions about nursing care. Managers should be able to recognize the value of other people's models or conceptual descriptions of the situation and use them to their best advantage. It is imperative that a good manager have a concept, theory, or model about worker motivation, for example, and how that affects the functioning of the organization.

8. *Recognizing your own influence on the organization.* Whether the nursing organization is a large one or a small one, the actions, the priorities, the decisions, even the attitudes and moods of the nurse manager affect the staff. The manager must realize that even apparently small, insignificant actions or comments can be interpreted by the staff to have more meaning than the manager may have intended. What may seem trivial to the nurse manager in the form of a hasty comment or a bit of careless information passed along may have a profound effect on the organization. The good nurse manager is aware and conscious of the fact that his or her actions can greatly influence the culture of the organization. The manager's influence filters down the organization to set values and norms. These evolve as a result of the manager's priorities. If a manager favors one given function within the organization, subordinates will quickly adjust and cater to that particular interest or function. For example, if a nurse manager is devoting much time to and sets a priority on scheduling and staffing, the subordinates perceive this as a valued aspect of the organization. This activity is perceived as one that the manager greatly values as opposed to, perhaps, interest in advances in nursing care. A wise manager then will allocate time as if he or she were setting priorities for the organization. If time is taken up with routine tasks or trivial tasks, these may be perceived by subordinates as valued issues that have priority for the manager and influence the development of the culture of the organization. The advent of microcomputers in nursing can free

nurse managers from many of the routine, repetitive tasks that previously have consumed a great deal of time. Staffing, scheduling, and aspects of budgeting can be computerized and free managers to pursue other goals.

9. *Dealing with a growing coalition.* Major changes in today's society and in attitudes toward work are significantly affecting the way a coalition manager deals with every day work. In our democratic society, people are seeking greater freedom and control in their lives, which extends to the workplace. It may be true that this increasing need for freedom and control in the workplace affects efficiency and productivity; however there is no way to regress to the era of the economic man when wages alone were expected to be sufficient motivation for workers. Even labor unions in the United States are becoming involved in issues of productivity and policy. These democratic influences within organizations mean that managers have to face coalitions not only from the top of their organizations but also from below. Nurses are a group who have needed and craved autonomy in the workplace for a long time. Nurses are beginning to achieve some autonomy in participative management, decision making, and in the form of primary nursing in many organizations. If the nurse manager is not already aware of the coalition of subordinates, they will make it known that they need their work to be more inherently satisfying, and to have same autonomy in carrying out their responsibilities.

Studies of what motivates people in excellent organizations have demonstrated that this need for autonomy and striving for management of the organization from below leads to a greater degree of satisfaction for employees. This satisfaction leads to increased motivation and decreased absenteeism and turnover. The work of Frederick Herzberg (1966) originally demonstrated through the concept of vertical job loading that people need a greater voice in decision making within their units of the organization. The work of Hackman and Oldham (1980) has also demonstrated that autonomy is a significant factor in increasing people's satisfaction and motivation on the job. The Magnet Hospital Study (1983), which related excellence in nursing to decreased turnover, found that Magnet hospitals offered a great degree of autonomy to their nursing staff. The second coalition that is growing and must be dealt with by the nursing organization is that from outside of the organization. Indeed, many top managers of large nursing organizations are becoming more like political leaders in their relationship to pressure groups of various kinds. The nurse manager at the level of chief executive officer will be paying more and more attention to the external roles of *liaison, spokesman, figurehead,* and *negotiator* in dealing with outside groups. The middle manager, meanwhile, will be called on to emphasize the *leader* role more and more and will adjust that leadership role to the changing complexity of coalitions within the organization.

10. *Using the management scientist or consultant.* Mintzberg urges in his final point for effective managing that the manager make use of the management scientist or consultant, and that he or she learn to work effectively in any comprehensive investigation of the organization. The consultant or expert should not be seen as someone who will come in and solve a particular problem for the nurse manager, but as someone with whom he or she can work through the sharing of information. The nurse manager may find it helpful to use a management consultant or specialist in health care management or nursing management to assist in strategic planning, financial management, and in developing sophisticated time scheduling systems, or computer-based management systems.

BASIC MANAGEMENT SKILLS

To function in the management roles and to be the effective manager discussed earlier in this chapter, a basic set of management skills must be learned by students of nursing management. They can be learned in a cognitive way through reading, lectures, and attendance at classes. They can be learned through simulation, for example role playing, and they can be learned on the job. Many nurse managers who have not had the advantage of a master's preparation in nursing management have learned their skills on the job. Indeed there are excellent nursing leaders in management positions today who were not privileged to have any formal management training, but perhaps because of their natural talents, have been effective managers.

However, if we plan to have effective nursing management in the most complex health care delivery system which has ever faced us in this nation, we cannot rely on the haphazard method of "the cream rising to the top" or "survival of the fittest." Hoping that all nurse managers will receive enough on-the-job training to be effective in their work is not sufficient. Nurse managers must seize the opportunity to learn the basic skills necessary to be equal to other health care managers. Opportunities are open to nurses in many graduate programs in nursing administration. These opportunities to gain cognitive knowledge, role play, and have " on-the-job" experience in practicum settings in nursing administration are becoming increasingly available across the country. What then are the basic skills viewed as crucial for a manager to achieve? Mintzberg has identified the following eight skills as crucial:

1. *Peer skills.* Nurse managers must be able to communicate with equals both on a formal and an informal basis. They need an extensive network of contacts within the organization and must have the ability to *negotiate: to trade in time and resources.* What are commonly thought of as political skills are important for the nurse manager. Those skills that are associated with managing conflict in large bureaucratic organizations are an example. These skills can be learned, and many nurse managers have the opportunity to learn them in the university setting or in management development workshops. Indeed, the teachers of nurse managers should use the potential for development of good peer skills in programs in nursing management.

2. *Leadership skills.* Good leadership skills require that nurse managers be able to motivate employees to deal with problems of *authority* and *dependence.* The development of leadership skills is one that has been addressed in nursing programs. Indeed, students of nursing, in both graduate and undergraduate programs, have been offered courses in leadership. However, Mintzberg states that, "Leadership, like swimming, cannot be learned by reading about it. Leadership skills are so closely related to the innate personality that it may be difficult to effect really significant change in a classroom" (1973, p. 190). Not all managers will be capable of the *transforming* leadership described in Chapter 3.

3. *Conflict resolution skills.* Conflict resolution is a style of interpersonal mediation between conflicting groups or individuals. It would be defined as Mintzberg's *disturbance handler* role of the manager. In performing conflict res-

olution, the manager is functioning under stress. Mintzberg believes that the manager can be trained to function
under the psychological stress that is present in the role
of negotiator or disturbance handler. Role-playing techniques and simulations may be helpful in training managers in good conflict resolution skills. The use of video-
tapes and playbacks is a good technique for students in
learning conflict resolution skills.

4. *Information processing skills.* The nurse manager must
learn how to disseminate information, express ideas effectively, and speak formally as a representative of the
organization. However, many nurse managers are not
trained to extract the unstructured, undocumented information that comes to the manager's hands and that is
often sought by them. The ability to analyze data is essential to today's nurse manager. A good foundation in
data analysis can be learned through rigorous nursing
research courses. Nurse managers must also have good
verbal skills. The telephone, scheduled and unscheduled
meetings, and tours of the facility are important sources
of contact and communication for the manager. Of course,
mail is also a source of communication and a manager must
know how to communicate in writing as well. Indeed, in
the age of tremendous information increase, the skill of
writing concisely and informatively is an invaluable one.
Information processing skills can be learned through formal education and through practice.

5. *Skills in decision making under ambiguity.* Many of the
nurse manager's decisions will be made in an unstructured
rather than in a structured situation. Indeed, in many
cases the nurse manager must first decide *when* a decision
must be made, then diagnose the situation and plan for
an approach to it. Students may be taught decision-making processes in nursing management courses that tend
to deal with the relatively routine and structured. In real
life, managers make decisions in times of uncertainty and
ambiguity. The gap between decision making in the rational, structured situations of the classroom versus the
reality of the workplace is large. Of course, it is worthwhile for the nurse manager to understand the process of
rational decision making. These studies will perhaps improve the manager's skills in decision making under ambiguity. However, we must also be attentive to the decision-making processes that the manager faces in the real
management situation. The skills needed for decision mak-

ing are considered of such importance that Chapter 6 is devoted to decision making in the nursing organization.

6. *Resource allocation.* Mintzberg states that learning to allocate resources is a skill that is not taught in many graduate programs in management. Although concepts and theories of staffing, scheduling, and patient classification may be presented, the nurse manager must learn to decide and choose among competing resource demands. • The first resource the manager must learn to allocate is his or her own time. Indeed the area of time management is so important that entire management development courses and workshops may be devoted to it. As well as managing their own time, nurse managers must learn how to determine what work subordinates must do and what kind of time allocation is expected of them. The allocation of *human resources* and *fiscal resources* are crucial skills for nurse managers, especially in this time of scarce resources. Courses in fiscal management and human resource management can teach these skills to the potential nurse manager. These two crucial elements form the basis of this text and Part II is entirely devoted to fiscal management in the nursing organization.

7. *Entrepreneurial skills.* The set of skills required of the entrepreneurial manager involves the ability to search for problems and opportunities for controlled change in the organization. Risk taking, innovation, and creativity are some of the skills of the entrepreneurial manager. For nurse managers to be good entrepreneurial managers, they must function in a climate that encourages the use of these skills. This climate of innovation and planned change is created by the chief executive officer of the organization and filters down to each department. A climate where creativity and innovation are rewarded rather than stifled helps to breed organizational excellence. Rosabeth Moss Kantor, in her book *The Change Masters* (1983, pp. 35–36), states that the skills needed to manage effectively in innovation-stimulating environments are:

• Power skills—skills in persuading others to invest information, support, and resources in new initiatives
• The ability to manage problems associated with greater use of teams and employee participation
• An understanding of how change is designed and constructed in an organization

8. *Introspection.* Nurse managers should thoroughly understand the job and be sensitive to their own impact on the
organization. Managers should also learn to look within
themselves and analyze the role before taking action. Introspection can be learned by nurse managers through
management training programs. Many self-development
tools exist for excellent training in the developmment of
self-awareness in the management role. Nurse managers
must have introspective skills to understand themselves
and the leadership role before they are challenged by the
complexities of human resource and fiscal resource management. The skills outlined previously can be developed
by nurse managers both in graduate programs in nursing
administration and in nursing management development
programs offered as continuing education. It should be
remembered, however, that even with education and
development not everyone can be or should be a nurse
manager.

> Successful managers are likely to demonstrate special
> ability to operate in peer relationships, to lead others
> in subordinate relationships, to resolve interpersonal
> and decisional conflicts, communicate in the verbal me-
> dia, to make complex interrelated decisions, to allocate
> resources (including their own time), and to innovate.
> (Mintzberg, 1973, p. 195)

Nurse managers at the executive and middle levels of the
organization must begin to identify the management potential within the organization and to groom those nurses with potential for management positions. This can be done through management development programs and by providing opportunities for
advanced education and career mobility for potential managers.
Only when we begin to identify those nurses with the *special
skills* necessary for nursing management will we improve the
pool of nurses from which we draw our managers and no longer
rely on self-selection and moving up through the ranks, as the
basis for development of nurse managers.

ACKNOWLEDGMENT

Much of the material for this chapter comes from *The Nature of Managerial Work* (1973) by Henry Mintzberg, with permission from Harper & Row, Publishers.

REFERENCES AND BIBLIOGRAPHY

Barnard, C.I. *The functions of the executive* (30th ed.). Cambridge, Mass.: Harvard University Press, 1968.

Brooten, D. *Managerial leadership in nursing.* Philadelphia: Lippincott, 1984.

Burns, J. McG. *Leadership.* New York: Harper & Row, Pub., 1978.

Hackman, J.R., & Oldham, G.R. *Work redesign.* Reading, Mass.: Addison-Wesley, 1980.

Herzberg, F. *Works and the nature of man.* Cleveland: World, 1966.

Kantor, R.M. *The change masters.* New York: Simon and Schuster, 1983.

McClure, M., Poulin, M., Sovie, M., & Wandelt, M. *Magnet hospitals.* Kansas City, Mo: American Nurses Association, 1983.

Mintzberg, H. *The nature of managerial work.* New York: Harper & Row, Pub., 1973.

Peters, T., & Waterman, R., Jr. *In search of excellence.* New York: Harper & Row, Pub., 1982.

CHAPTER 3

The Individual in the Nursing Organization

In the preceding chapters we have investigated the concept of the organization as an open system that interacts with its environment, with a complex transformation process requiring a good fit between the formal organizational structure, the informal structure, the task of the organization, and the individual. The individual is by far the most important element in any organization. Without people nothing can happen—indeed there can be no organization. It is increasingly recognized in many sectors of American industry that the difference between the excellent organization and the mediocre organization is the motivation of the individual in that organization. Nursing organizations are no exception, as the 1983 American Academy of Nursing Study on retention, *Magnet Hospitals*, demonstrated. The Magnet hospitals study showed that the difference between *their* retention and turnover rates and those of other hospitals was based on the motivation of the nursing staff. But how are employees motivated? Indeed, can one person motivate another? What makes one nurse a highly motivated and creative member of the nursing staff and another indifferent or mediocre? Questions regarding motivation of the individual at work are complex. We will explore the theories that will help to unravel some of these complexities for the nurse manager who faces the especially difficult task of motivating the professional employee.

MOTIVATION

For at least the first half of this century, American management was strongly influenced by the work of Frederick Taylor and his "Scientific Management Method" (Taylor, 1911). The Taylor influence is still evident in many sectors of American industry. Scientific management is premised on increasing productivity by reducing work to its simplest elements through techniques such as *time and motion studies*. Nursing, along with much of American industry has been moving away from the kind of fractionalized work assignments that resulted from Taylorism. In nursing, the *functional* nursing assignment has been replaced by concepts such as total patient care and primary nursing. In industry, the demoralizing effects of assembly line work have been recognized, and efforts have been made in many sectors to create more meaningful units of work. Taylor's philosophy permeated the early industrial era in America. The worker was viewed as essentially motivated by economic factors. Producing the most efficient worker was seen as being beneficial both to management and to the individual worker. For management, reducing work to its simplest elements allowed for greater productivity. For the worker, increasing the output resulted in an increase in monetary rewards.

A broader understanding of the needs of the worker, both professional and nonprofessional, began to evolve with the now famous *Hawthorne studies*. These studies, which were conducted at the Hawthorne Plant of the Western Electric Factory, demonstrated that workers were motivated by elements much more complex than extrinsic rewards, such as pay or physical conditions alone. The studies at the Hawthorne plant were conducted over a series of years and began with experiments to find out what the quality and the quantity of light should be to produce the most efficiency in a group of industrial workers. The Hawthorne studies became illuminating themselves when experimenters discovered that whether lighting was increased or decreased, whether workers used the same illumination intensity, or whether the intensity was varied in the control groups, production *increased* in both the experimental and the control groups. The increase in production was about the same in both groups. This effect has become known in research as the *Hawthorne effect*. Several groups of experimental illumination changes produced the same kinds of findings. Whether the group was the experimental group or the control group, there was no appreciable difference between the groups. These findings had the researchers very puzzled. They thought perhaps one difficulty in their study was trying to study a single variable such as illumination when there were many uncontrolled variables in the situation.

But as Roethlisberger and Dickson (1941) point out:

> A few of the tough minded experimenters already were beginning to suspect their basic ideas and assumptions with regard to human motivation. It occurred to them that the trouble was not so much with the results or the subjects as it was with the notion regarding the way their subjects were supposed to behave—the notion of a simple cause and effect, direct relationship between certain physical changes in the workers' environment and the responses of the workers to these changes. Such a notion completely ignored the human meaning of these changes to the people who were subjected to them. (Roethlisberger, 1941, p. 31)

As a result of the illumination research and further research studies in the bank wiring observation room, the Hawthorne researchers found that *peer groups, social interaction,* and *attention from management* played a significant role in worker motivation. The analysis of the Hawthorne studies in the 1940s began a new era in the management of human resources. Management began to appreciate that employees were more than mere pawns in an industrial machine. The age of Taylorism began to decline and a view of the worker as a *social being,* requiring intrinsic as well as extrinsic rewards from the work, came to influence motivation theory.

Abraham Maslow's hierarchy of needs has formed the basis for many of the motivation theories that have evolved since the Hawthorne studies. Table 3–1 illustrates Maslow's hierarchy of needs as it relates to the development of human resources theory. Classical theories, such as McGregor's Theory X and Theory Y (1960) and Herzberg's Motivation–Hygiene Theory (1966), are built on Maslow's framework. As Table 3–1 illustrates, the lower order needs can be equated with the rise of Taylorism and the focus on the economic and security needs of the individual. The social needs of the individual, which were discovered at the time of the Hawthorne studies, equate with Maslow's next level of need, for belonging and socialization. McGregor, Herzberg, and some later theorists focus on the intrinsic rewards from the work itself, which meet the higher order of needs for esteem and self-actualization.

TABLE 3-1. A CONCEPTUALIZATION OF THE DEVELOPMENT OF HUMAN
RESOURCES THEORY

Maslow's Needs Hierarchy	Concepts Regarding Work Motivation
Need for valued rewards	*Cognitive Man* Expectancy Theory Vroom 1980s–1990s
Need for esteem/self-actualization	*Psychological Man* Maslow, Herzberg, McGregor, Hackman & Oldham 1960s–1980s
Need for belonging/recognition	*Social Man* Hawthorne studies, Homans 1940s–1960s
Need for safety/security	*Economic Man* Taylor 1900s–1940s

McGregor's Theory

After the Hawthorne studies, work by theorists such as Abraham
Maslow, Douglas McGregor, and Chris Argyris began to reshape
the notion of what motivates people at work. The newer and
more complex view of the nature of people at work was explained
in Douglas McGregor's Theory X and Theory Y (McGregor, 1960).
McGregor proposed that there were basically two sets of managerial assumptions about the nature of the worker. In Theory
X, he proposed that managers held what might be thought of as
a traditional view of the worker as basically indolent, lazy, and
lacking in ambition.

Theory X views the worker as self-centered, resisting change,
basically gullible, and not very bright. The Theory X manager
would use the "carrot and stick," autocratic approach to managing
the subordinate workers. McGregor then proposed a set of managerial assumptions which he labeled Theory Y. The Theory Y
assumptions were the embodiment of the newer view of people
at work that was evolving in the 1960s and was built on the
Hawthorne studies, the work of Maslow, and others. Theory Y
proposes that people are primarily self-motivated and self-con-
trolled, and that if given a chance employees will integrate their
goals with those of the organization. People are seen as basically

self-motivated, interested in achievement, and striving to be mature. A manager assuming a Theory Y stance would have a broader base of power and a more democratic organization than a manager espousing Theory X. McGregor's influence can be seen in the growth of the concept of participative management.

Herzberg's Theory

Herzberg's Motivation–Hygiene theory grew out of research conducted in the late 1950s and early 1960s. In studies of accountants, engineers, and other professionals, Herzberg developed his two-factor theory (Herzberg, 1966). The *motivators* or *satisfiers*, described by Herzberg, are those elements that are intrinsic in the work itself such as recognition, achievement, responsibility, advancement, personal growth, and confidence.

The *hygiene factors*, or dissatisfiers, are those extrinsic elements such as salary, company policies, work environment, relationships with peers, and relationships with subordinates and supervisors (Table 3–2). When studying Herzberg's theory one must not assume that the opposite of dissatisfaction is satisfaction. On the contrary, Herzberg points out that a lack of hygiene factors will lead to dissatisfaction; however, when hygiene factors are gratified they will lead to a lack of dissatisfaction, rather than to satisfaction. When the motivating factors described by Herzberg are gratified they will lead to job satisfaction. Herzberg proposed principles of *vertical job loading* to increase the motivators or the satisfiers for the worker. Table 3–3 describes vertical job loading techniques aimed at giving workers more autonomy and responsibility.

TABLE 3–2. THE ELEMENTS OF HERZBERG'S TWO-FACTOR THEORY OF MOTIVATION

Dissatisfaction or Hygiene Factors	Satisfaction or Motivating Factors
Company policy and administration	Achievement
Supervision (technical)	Recognition for achievement
Relationships with supervisor	Work itself
Work conditions	Responsibility
Salary	Advancement or growth
Relationships with peers	
Status and security	

TABLE 3–3. VERTICAL JOB TRADING PRINCIPLES

Principle	Motivator
Remove some controls	Responsibility, achievement
Increase accountability for own work	Responsibility, recognition
Create natural units of work	Responsibility, achievement, recognition
Increase worker's autonomy	Responsibility, achievement, recognition
Feedback directly to worker	Recognition
Introduce new, more difficult, or specialized tasks	Growth, learning
Allow individuals to become experts or specialists	Responsibility, growth, advancement

NEWER CONCEPTS IN MOTIVATION THEORY

Job Diagnostic Model

Hackman and Oldham's *Job Characteristic Theory* (Hackman and Oldham, 1979) builds on the work of theorists, such as Herzberg, but has the advantage of greater specificity in examining a particular individual's job in detail. Guidelines for job design intervention are explicit and include such tools as the Job Diagnostic Survey and the Job Rating Form, which assist in diagnosing the specific elements of a job that need improvement. The Job Diagnostic model proposes that positive work outcomes, such as high motivation, satisfaction, and low absenteeism and turn-over, are the result of critical psychological states. The *critical psychological states* are arrived at through the proper balance of five core job dimensions: *skill variety, task identity, task significance, autonomy,* and *feedback.*

A conceptualization of the model is presented in Figure 3–1. Hackman and Oldham's model is based on the notion of building into jobs those elements that most contribute to high motivation and performance, recognizing that different people will respond differently to the same job. Two moderating influences on the core job dimensions are (1) the individual's need for personal growth and (2) the satisfaction of the employee with the work context i.e., hygiene factors such as pay and job security. Figure 3–1 illustrates that the *core job dimensions* influence a person's critical psychological states, which in turn influence the personal outcomes. Based on the Job Characteristics theory, Hackman and Oldham developed a method of measuring the motivating potential of an individual job. The *Motivating Potential Score,* or MPS, is computed as illustrated in Figure 3–2. Hackman and Oldham caution that not everyone benefits from a job with a high

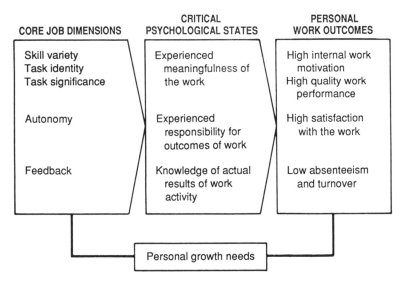

Figure 3–1. The Hackman–Oldham Job Characteristics model. (*From Hackman and Oldham. Work Redesign, 1980, Addison-Wesley, Reading, Massachusetts. Reprinted with permission.*)

motivating potential score. Individuals who have a strong need for growth and accomplishment will respond well, whereas individuals without these strong needs may find an enriched job anxiety provoking and may feel out of their depth.

In a survey of 25 nurses in staff nurse positions, Kirsch (1984) found that the staff nurses unanimously rated their jobs as high in skill variety, task identity, and task significance. Most nurse managers would agree that these dimensions typify the role of the staff nurse.

Not unexpectedly, however, the dimensions of autonomy and feedback were not as clearly present in the majority of staff nurse positions. Of the 25 nurses surveyed, 20 rated their jobs as low in autonomy and 18 rated them as low in feedback. Thus the two dimensions most most important for a high MPS score are the areas where staff nurse positions may be lacking.

The Hackman–Oldham model for job diagnosis provides a set of *change principles*, which can be used as guides for im-

$$\text{Motivating Potential Score (MPS)} = \frac{\text{Skill Variety} + \text{Task Variety} + \text{Task Significance}}{3} \times \text{Autonomy} \times \text{Feedback}$$

Figure 3–2. Calculating the motivating potential score (MPS) from the job diagnostic survey.

proving low scores in any of the five core job dimensions. Table 3–4 presents the *Change Principles*. A low score in skill variety and task identity, for instance, would be changed by combining tasks; that is, taking fractionalized job elements and combining them into a meaningful unit of work. Task identity and task significance can be increased by forming natural work units, that is, distributing work based on experience, training, and efficiency to create equity among individual work loads. The areas that may be of greatest concern for the nurse manager appear to be the dimensions of autonomy and feedback. As can be seen by the change principles in Table 3–4, these dimensions can be increased by improving client relationships, vertical loading, and opening feedback channels. The concept of vertical loading involves giving the employees some of the responsibilities and controls usually reserved for management. Staff nurses, for example, could decide on management of their own time and have some scheduling responsibilities.

A sharing of financial aspects of the nursing organization, with some input into budgeting decisions, is another example of vertical loading that could increase autonomy. A voice in some of the management decisions that affect their work lives can be of great help in increasing autonomy in a nursing staff and thereby increasing motivation.

The positive effects of a high feedback score can be achieved through improving client relationships in ways that would allow the staff nurse to receive direct feedback from the patient regarding the quality of care received. This can be done through formal procedures that are frequent and relevant to care being rendered to specific patients. Direct feedback from patients gives each staff nurse responsibility for quality control, and thus opens feedback channels between patient and nurse. Feedback channels from the work itself can be enhanced in this way. Feedback re-

TABLE 3–4. CHANGE PRINCIPLES FOR USE WITH THE JOB DIAGNOSTIC MODEL

Change Principles	Skill Variety	Tasks Identity	Tasks Significance	Autonomy	Feedback
Combining tasks	X	X			
Forming natural work units		X	X		
Establishing client relationships	X				X
Vertical loading				X	X
Opening feedback channels					X

garding job performance should go along with improved patient feedback. Staff nurses should receive clear information about their performance at frequent and regular intervals, including positive as well as negative aspects of job performance. Nursing, by its very nature, offers a great many intrinsic rewards, i.e., rewards from the work itself. The Hackman–Oldham model offers a way to examine a job, diagnose its deficiencies, and apply principles of change to increase these intrinsic rewards, which lead to greater motivation (Hackman and Oldham, 1979).

Expectancy Theory

The newest approach to the study of motivation in organizations is *Expectancy Theory*. Nadler, Tushman, and Hatvany (1982) point out that expectancy theory is based on a set of specific assumptions about the causes of behavior in organizations. First, it is assumed that behavior is determined by a combination of forces in the individual and forces in the environment. Neither the individual nor the environment alone determines behavior in this view. It assumes that people come into organizations with a past psychological and developmental history that gives them a unique set of needs, or ways of looking at the world, and expectations about how an organization will treat them. Second, people make decisions about their own behavior in organizations. This assumption holds that people make conscious decisions about their behavior in organizations. Individuals make decisions about coming to work, staying at work, and other ways of being a member of the organization. They also make decisions about the amount of effort they will direct toward performing their jobs. The third assumption made by the expectancy theory is that different people have different needs, desires, and goals. This assumption holds that individuals differ in what kinds of rewards they desire. The expectancy theory assumes that these differences are not random, that they can be examined systematically, and that by understanding these differences, we can meet individual needs.

The fourth assumption made by the expectancy theory is that people make decisions among alternative plans of behavior, based on their perceptions or expectancies of the degree to which a given behavior will lead to a desired outcome. In other words, people tend to do those things that they see as leading to rewards that they desire, and avoid doing those things that they see as leading to rewards or outcomes that are not desired.

The expectancy theory poses a cognitive approach to the management of individual behavior in organizations. It supposes that people come into organizations with their own needs and conceptualizations to make decisions about how they will behave *consciously*. The reliance of the model on the concept of rational decision making does raise some questions about its validity.

> The model is based on the assumption that individuals make very rational decisions after a thorough exploration of all the available alternatives and on weighing the possible outcomes of these alternatives. When we talk to or observe individuals, however, we find that their decision processes are frequently less thorough. People often stop considering alternative behavioral plans when they find one that is at least moderately satisfying, even though more rewarding plans remain to be examined. (Nadler, Tushman, and Hatvany, 1982, pp. 104–105)

Even with the cautions about the limitations of the model, it can be useful to the manager in determining valid ways of motivating their staff. Figure 3–3 presents a *basic motivation-behavior sequence*. The sequence demonstrates motivation as the force on the individual to expend effort. Motivation leads to an observed level of effort by the individual. Performance results from the level of effort put forth by the individual and the skills and abilities that the individual brings to the work situation. As a result of the performance, the individual gains certain outcomes. The expected outcomes are not always forthcoming after performance. The performance–reward cycle occurs time after time and the actual rewards resulting from a performance provide information that influences the individual's perception and motivation for the future.

The kinds of outcomes or rewards a person values fall into two categories. First, the individual obtains rewards from the organizational environment. A certain level of performance in-

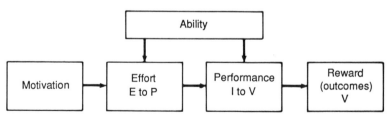

Motivation results from:
   E–Effort to performance expectancies
   V–Perceived valence or value of outcomes
   I–Correlation of performance to outcome expectancies

Figure 3–3. The motivation–behavior sequence proposed in expectancy theory. *(From Nadler and Lawler. In Hackman and Lawler, Perspectives on Behavior in Organizations, McGraw-Hill, 1977. Reprinted with permission.)*

dicates that an individual will receive positive or negative rewards from supervisors, co-workers, and the formal reward system of an organization. These kinds of rewards would be classified as extrinsic rewards, that is, coming from outside of the individual, from organizational sources. A second source of rewards for the individual are those characterized as intrinsic rewards. These are rewards from the work itself and include feelings of accomplishment, achievement, and personal worth. They would be equated with Herzberg's motivators or satisfiers and Maslow's higher order of needs.

The expectancy theory bases the motivation–behavior sequence on the kind of extrinsic and intrinsic rewards that the individual will come to expect from a given performance in an organization. Nadler, Hackman, and Lawler point out that after more than 50 studies to test the validity of the expectancy theory, "the theory correctly predicts that the leads about the outcomes associated with performance (expectancy) will be better predictors of performance than will feelings about job satisfaction since expectancies are the critical causes of performance and satisfaction is not" (1982, p. 104).* What then are the implications for managers from the findings related to the expectancy theory? To use the expectancy theory to increase motivation, the manager must diagnose both the person and the organizational environment. The manager must:

1. Find out what outcomes each employee values. This may be done through structured measurement and data collection and through observations of employees' reactions to rewards. It can be done simply by asking employees what kinds of rewards they would like to have for a given performance.
2. The manager must determine what kinds of behavior or performance he or she expects. It is essential that the managers clearly define the performance level expected of an employee to achieve a given reward.
3. The manager must make sure that the desired levels of performance are achievable by the employee. If a manager sets a level of performance that the employee feels is impossible to achieve, then the performance level is likely to be relatively low.
4. The manager must make sure that the desired rewards are clearly linked to the desired performances. If your

---

* A detailed discussion of expectancy theory, including the expectancy formula and questionnaires used to put expectancy theory into practice, is given in Appendix A.

employees value pay raises, then it must be clear what kinds of performances will lead to those merit increases. If your employees value career mobility, it must be clear what the performance must be to move up to the next step on the career ladder.

Having followed these guidelines, the manager should be careful that there are no conflicting expectancies set up in the organization's reward system. Nadler, Tushman, and Hatvany caution that "Motivation will only be high when people see a number of rewards associated with good performance and few negative outcomes" (1982, p. 106). The manager must also make sure that the rewards offered are big enough to initiate changes in motivation. If rewards are trivial in nature then they are apt to result in trivial increases in motivation. A final caution for the manager in using the expectancy theory: make sure that the reward system is equitable.

> Good performers should see that they get more desired rewards than do poor performers, and others in the system should see that also. Equity should not be confused with a system of equality, where all are rewarded equally with no regard for their performance. A system of equality is guaranteed to produce low motivation. (Nadler, Hackman, and Lawler, 1979, p. 106)

REWARDS SYSTEMS

The expectancy theory demonstrates that the desired outcomes expected by employees for a given performance can be either extrinsic or intrinsic rewards. In reality, most nurse middle managers may have little control over extrinsic rewards systems in their organizations. Monetary rewards such as salary, fringe benefits, and merit pay increases, are often items that are negotiated in a labor contract. Other types of extrinsic rewards that deal with promotion or career mobility may be in the jurisdiction of nurse middle managers and can be influenced by them. The discussion of reward systems then, will concentrate on the kinds of rewards most middle managers can make. Peters and Waterman, in their book, *In Search of Excellence* (1982), have demonstrated that most of the excellent corporations in America make great use of nonmonetary rewards. Nonmonetary rewards can be used to great advantage by nurse middle managers.

The clever use of nonmonetary rewards can motivate nursing staff. Observations have shown that most nurse managers know very little about the tremendous benefits of positive reinforcement; they may even consider it undignified or unprofessional to give positive reinforcement. *Positive reinforcement* is one of the easiest nonmonetary kinds of rewards a manager can give to a staff member. The manager must understand how to give positive reinforcement. There are several simple schemes and approaches outlined by Peters and Waterman (1982, p. 70) for the giving of positive reinforcement. First, positive reinforcement must be *specific*, relevant to a particular performance. In other words, a general kind of "you're doing a good job" is not the kind of positive reinforcement we are discussing. Rather, a manager should congratulate a particular goal reached for a particular job well done. It must be very specific. Second, positive reinforcement should have *immediacy*. The reinforcement should come as close to the event as possible, not many weeks later.

An example of immediacy is given in this quote from *In Search of Excellence:*

> Late one evening, a scientist rushed into the president's office with a working prototype of a new design that the company had been working on for many years; the president was dumbfounded at the elegance of the solution and he was bemused about how to reward it. He bent forward in his chair, rummaged through most of the drawers in his desk, and he found something. He leaned over the desk and gave it to the scientist "Here." In his hands was a banana, the only reward he could immediately put his hands on. From that point on the small gold banana pin has been the highest allocade for scientific achievement at Foxborough. (Peters and Waterman, 1982, pp. 70–71)

Third, the reward–feedback system should have *achievability*. As in the expectancy theory, we caution here that managers must set achievable levels of performance and that they must reward the small achievements or goals reached as well as the big ones. The intangible effect of attention from management is a reward in itself. It is well known from the Hawthorne studies that attention from management can cause an increase in productivity. This phenomenon, termed the Hawthorne effect, proved that attention from management is a reward in itself.

Fourth, rewards should be *unpredictable* and *intermittent*. Frequent and expected rewards tend to lose their value. The yearly merit increase or bonus is not a reward. It is expected and it is frequent, and it begins to lose its value for employees. Also, the kind of merit increase that comes yearly and automatically does not have equity as its base, but equality. As cautioned in the discussion on the expectancy theory, equality causes rewards to lose their value.

The giving of small, nonmonetary rewards with immediacy requires nurse managers who, in Mintzberg's words "tour their organization." If a nurse manager goes out, walks around the organization and sees what is going on, he or she can give small verbal rewards on the spot. Small, symbolic rewards can be kept less political than big, important awards, where committees decide who is selected for an annual award such as the best Cardiac Nurse of the Year. We must understand in rewarding individuals that people compare themselves to their peers and *not* to the absolute standards of achievement that we may outline on performance evaluation forms. They want to know if other units are doing better than theirs, and how are their peers doing. These observations are constantly made by one employee about another as a way of assessing progress.

Small, nonmonetary rewards, given by managers to staff, may be thought of as a form of feedback. In the discussion of motivation it was shown that many staff nurse jobs are lacking in feedback as one of the chief motivating factors. This seems a fairly simple way for nurse managers to begin to increase the motivation of their staff; using the imaginative nonmonetary rewards that are at their discretion as a form of feedback can increase motivation significantly.

Autonomy was also indicated as an essential ingredient in increasing motivation in the Hackman–Oldham model. Peters and Waterman support concern about the need for employees to have control over their destinies. They point out that social psychology research has shown that if people think that they have even a modest control over their destinies, they persist at tasks, they do better at them, and they become committed to them. This phenomenon has been termed the *illusion of control* by social psychologists (Peters and Waterman, 1982, pp. 80–81). The illusion of control ties in with research, which indicates that autonomy and feedback were the greatest single motivators for a group of staff nursing jobs (Kirsch, 1984). The Magnet hospital study (1983) also reinforces these findings, demonstrating that nurse satisfaction and decreased absenteeism and turnover were highly related to the autonomy that nurses in this study perceived themselves to have. If we have a bit more discretion or autonomy in our work lives, we have a much bigger commitment to whatever it is that we are doing. Allowing as much autonomy as possible and pushing authority as far down the ladder as we possibly can will lead to a greater commitment and motivation of staff.

We like to think of ourselves as winners. The lesson that the excellent companies have to teach is that there is no reason why we can't design systems that continually reinforce this notion; most of their people are made to feel that they are winners. *Their populations are distributed around the normal curve, just like any other large population, but the difference is that their systems reinforce degrees of winning rather than degrees of losing* (emphasis added). (Peters and Waterman, 1982, p. 57)

We can design nursing organizations and their reward systems to reinforce the notion that most people think of themselves as winners. We can design systems that reinforce degrees of winning, rather than degrees of losing by setting realistic goals for achievement and by giving frequent, positive reinforcement. The small, nonmonetary, verbal or symbolic reward pays off tremendously in terms of worker motivation and satisfaction. Nurse managers should think *excellence* and *achievable goals*, and *reward performance* in a way that is valued by their staff. These are the cardinal elements for a successful motivation–reward system for the nursing organization.

REFERENCES AND BIBLIOGRAPHY

Argyris, C. *Personality and organization.* New York: Harper & Row, Pub., 1957.

Fayol, H. *General and industrial administration.* London: Pitman & Sons, 1949.

Hackman, J.R., & Oldham, G.R. *Work redesign.* Reading, Mass.: Addison-Wesley, 1979.

Herzberg, F. *Work and the nature of man.* Cleveland: World, 1966.

Homans, G.C. *The human group.* New York: Harcourt Brace, 1950.

Kirsch, J. Application of a job diagnostic model to the motivation of staff. *Health Care Supervisor,* April, 1984.

Levinson, H. *The great jackass fallacy.* Boston: Harvard University Press, 1977.

Levinson, H. *Psychological man.* Cambridge, Mass.: The Levinson Institute, 1976.

Maslow, A.H. *Motivation and personality.* New York: Harper & Row, Pub., 1954.

McClure, M., Poulin, M., Sovie, M., & Wandelt, M. *Magnet hospitals.* Kansas City, Mo.: American Nurses Association, 1983.

McGregor, D. *The human side of enterprise.* New York: McGraw–Hill, 1960.

Nadler, D., Hackman, J.R., & Lawler, E.E. *Managing organizational behavior.* Boston: Little, Brown, 1979.

Nadler, D., Tushman, M., & Hatvany, N. *Managing organizations: Readings and cases.* Boston: Little, Brown, 1982.

Ouchi, W. *Theory Z.* Reading, Mass.: Addison-Wesley, 1981.

Peters, T., & Waterman, R.H. *In search of excellence.* New York: Harper & Row, Pub., 1982.

Roethlisberger, F., & Dickson, J. *Management and the worker.* Cambridge: Harvard University Press, 1939.

Taylor, F. *The principles of scientific management.* New York: Harper & Row, Pub., 1911.

Vroom, V. *Work and motivation.* New York: Wiley, 1964.

CHAPTER 4

Managing the Group in the Nursing Organization

Donna M. Costello-Nickitas

Ever since the now historic Hawthorne studies of the thirties and forties, the importance of the group in the workplace has not been doubted. The Hawthorne experience revealed that attention to workers, as well as conditions, impact on productivity. The social interaction that occurs between workers in group situations and between workers and managers can improve job satisfaction. Groups serve several functions within an organization. This chapter explores the nature, function, and impact of groups within the nursing organization, including (1) types of groups, (2) functions of groups, (3) power and politics of groups, (4) conflict and conflict resolution within groups, (5) labor relations as an example of conflict resolution, and (6) the nurse manager's role in collective bargaining.

The group experience can serve to satisfy personal and social needs as well as promote organizational objectives. How groups perform, their effectiveness and productivity, has many variations, from disastrous to excellent. A nurse manager has the ability to improve group productivity and work quality by understanding the relationship between the individual and the group. The two factors that affect this relationship are work group effectiveness, how well the group performs its tasks, and social influence, how groups are influenced by individuals. The extent to which individuals at work are affected by the group to which they belong will impact their job satisfaction and productivity.

GROUPS AND THE NURSING ORGANIZATION

Groups are subsystems of the organization. Although individuals may perform tasks, the majority of organizational work is performed by collections of people working together. Groups are "collections of two or more people interacting with each other and thinking of themselves as a unit" (Nadler, Hackman, and Lawler, 1979, p. 16).

Types of Groups

Within any organization there are a variety of groups that can exist. The functions and purposes of each group often go unnoticed because of their unique diversity in meeting organizational needs. Among the types of groups existing in nursing organizations are work groups, interdisciplinary teams, management groups, informal groups, and demographic groups.

Work Groups. These are groups of individuals on any particular unit who work together to provide a service or produce a product. A pediatric nursing unit or team, intravenous therapy nurses, or clinical nurse specialists are examples of work groups.

Interdisciplinary Teams. These are work groups with a short life span developed for a specific problem or task. A team is made up of diverse members with special expertise. An interdisciplinary health care team, consisting of a nurse, physician, social worker, and dietitian, might consider a particular patient's needs.

Management Groups. These are work groups that share responsibility for managing a unit or a group. This group is charged with making decisions that may effect policy, practice, personnel, and budget. Head nurses and supervisory committees are examples of management groups.

Informal Groups. These are groups that have no defined relationship to the overall structure and purpose of the organization, but have a shared interest in its goals and objectives. This group can be powerful when informally agreeing on what needs to be accomplished for the organization.

Demographic Groups. These are groups that share personal attributes such as age, race, gender, or ethnicity. The members of demographic groups may not interact with each other but they can serve as a powerful reference group for their members; for instance, the Gray Panthers, National Organization of Women, and the Black Nurses Association.

Functions of Groups in the Organization

Groups serve several functions for the organization and the individual. Specifically, groups can be comprised of individuals who are experts at accomplishing tasks that cannot be performed individually. Here, group members build simple tasks into complex structures. For the group to grow and develop in their tasks, the members can facilitate change by using the group as a vehicle for decision making. This allows for conflicting views to be expressed and considered. Vroom and Yetton's decision model stresses the importance of group involvement in the decision process. Group involvement results in the strongest commitment of subordinates to the implementation of the decision (Vroom and Yetton, 1973). Here, group discussion gives way to free exchange of ideas and a give-and-take among member viewpoints occurs. Because of this mutual exchange of ideas, social pressure toward conformity of thought and action can influence the individual behavior of group members. Group pressure leads to the organization control of individual behavior. By transmitting shared beliefs and values to new members, the organization's rules and regulations are perpetuated. This is intended to lead to increased organizational success and stability.

The success of an organization is dependent on the individuals who are its members. Belonging to a group within an organization satisfies important individual needs. Individuals have strong needs for affiliation and acceptance by group members. The group experience allows the individual to gain self-awareness and confidence in performing tasks. The help, knowledge, and reward that is obtained from group work sometimes is not accessible through individual effort. Group membership can help individuals achieve both personal and organizational goals. How an individual relates to a group is key to his or her survival and success in the organization. Nurse managers must consider individuals' needs and abilities and attempt to identify a group that can benefit both the individual and the organization. Ultimately, a good match between an individual and a group can improve job satisfaction and reduce turnover, absenteeism, and lateness. Nurse managers can develop an effective work group by matching the individual to a group through a successful job interview—assigning the individual to an experienced nurse to serve as perceptor and maintaining personal contact and follow-up. This personal contact helps to lessen the feelings of isolation an individual may experience when first exposed to the organization.

Social Intensity

As a new member of the work group, the individual quickly encounters *the social influence* from its members. This social influence of groups on individual members is measured by something called social intensity. "Social intensity determines how much of an effect the group is likely to have on its members and on the functioning of the broader organization" (Nadler, Hackman, and Lawler, 1979, p. 106).

The level of social intensity for a group can be measured on a scale from low to high. Nadler, Hackman, and Lawler illustrate the continuum of social intensity by identifying three groups in the organization: reference groups (low end), co-acting groups (middle), and traditional groups (high end). The intensity of group interaction has great significance to group members and influences their values and beliefs.

Reference Groups. This refers to individuals who use the group as a point of reference for validating their beliefs or attitudes or assessing their level of performance or skill. These individuals may not have direct contact with the group but their membership is determined by their personal attributes, such as age, race, ethnic or religious background, or organization/professional affiliation.

Co-Acting Groups. This refers to individuals who have face-to-face contact and interact informally. These individuals do not work together on a common group goal or task. They perform individual tasks in the presence of other individuals and have the same supervisor. Members of co-acting groups do not have strong social bonds since they do not depend on each other for coordinate tasks. Primary nursing illustrates how individuals can work side by side with others and still have their own assignment.

Traditional Groups. This refers to individuals who create their own history and set of traditions, values, and beliefs over time that are eventually accepted by the group. Here, individuals work together, share time together, and value the group as an important part of their lives.

Work groups, such as any nursing care unit, management or critical care team, can be called a traditional group. Members know their duties and perform them accordingly. There are clear relationships with strong influence on certain behaviors and attitudes toward group activities.

As technology advances and human interaction in the workplace is identified as an essential for productivity, nurse managers much understand the benefits and risks of high social intensity. A group that is high in social intensity places pressure on its members to conform. Conformity leads to control over members' behavior and performance by peers. Members care about what their peers think of them. Interpersonal awards and acceptance by peers are important group values. Because peer pressure can lead to enforcement of group goals rather than organizational goals, nurse managers must assess the social intensity of their groups. Too much social influence from a group can render it ineffective in providing a service by performing tasks inadequately. The group effort becomes invested in protecting its self-interests as opposed to promoting organizational goals.

High social intensity induces cooperation and builds barriers to protect group members from organizational threats such as changes in organization policies, rules, and regulations. When a group acts synergistically to accomplish its task, as assembly effect develops. An assembly effect is a unique product of group members acting together (Collins and Guetzkow, 1964). The outcome of members working together creates a unique energy resulting in sustained morale and economic soundness for the organization. However, the assembly effect of groups can exert powerful influences on members' behavior and result in a *group think*. Each member of the group becomes engrossed in the group's values, beliefs, and norms, so that organizational tasks have low priority. The impact of group think on organizational development and task accomplishment can be devastating. The group loses its objectivity by reinforcing its values and beliefs, regardless of whether these values and beliefs are valid.

To overcome the negative effects of group think on organizational goals, the nurse manager can clarify and instill the value system of the organization. Each organization creates a basic philosophy or belief system that promotes its goals and objectives. Peters and Waterman (1982, p. 285) suggest that the dominant beliefs of excellent companies instill the basic values of:

- A belief in being the best
- A belief in the importance of the details of execution, the nuts and bolts of doing the job well
- A belief in the importance of people as individuals
- A belief in superior quality and service

• A belief in the importance of informality to enhance communication

The promotion and protection of these organizational values
can enhance the relationship between the manager and the members of the group. The manager creates an environment where
excellence in performance has to do with members being motivated by organizational values. The values of care, compassion,
and commitment to excellence can promote a positive self-image
and enhance members' productivity. These values help to shape
members' behavior and provide positive reinforcement for work
well done.

POWER AND POLITICS

Implications for Groups

To maintain the values and goals of the organization, the nurse
manager must cultivate and maintain political alliances. By using
power and politics to influence group decisions and actions, the
nurse manager builds unity, strength, and cohesiveness. Politics
is defined as any behavior used by an organizational member or
group that is self-serving (Robbins, 1976). Politics is functional
when the behavior used assists in the attainment of organizational
goals. It is dysfunctional when it hinders these goals. Political
behavior involves the use of power and authority. Power is the
potential of one individual or group to influence the behavior of
another. Power is the basic energy needed to initiate and sustain
action; the capacity to translate intention into reality and sustain
it (Bennis and Nanus, 1985, p. 17). Authority is the legal power
or the right to act. Authority, or legal power, comes with an
appointed position in an organization, i.e., chief executive officer,
director of nursing, assistant director, and others. It is this authority of position that determines an individual's responsibility,
accountability, and liability. Authority is an essential ingredient
underlying the role of a manager. Managers are responsible to
be knowledgeable about and function within the established
boundaries of their authority within the organization. A successful manager will use the political behaviors of power and authority
to control what will happen when she or he acts to get something
done.

By understanding political behavior, the nurse manager can
interpret organizational structures. This seems logical, since the
structures of power, decision making, and communication are
used by the manager to further organizational goals. Formal or-

ganizational structures reduce or eliminate uncertainty, thus reducing political behavior. However, members of the organization find ways of penetrating these structures to develop informal networks. A network functions as an informal structure where information, influence, and affect is exchanged. Nadler, Hackman, and Lawler (1979) define *information* as the flow of information between individuals or groups, *influence* as the ability of one individual or group to induce behavior in another, and *affect* as the positive or negative feelings that individuals or groups have toward each other.

Cliques and Coalitions: Consequences of Group Networks

As the network exchanges information, influence, and affect, linkages are made between groups in the organization. The groups that evolve from these linkages are called cliques and coalitions. Cliques are basic building blocks of political structures (Nadler, Hackman, and Lawler, 1979). They have their own norms for influencing the behavior of members. Cliques tend to work on certain organizational issues, establishing cooperative action strategies. When a number of cliques come together to take cooperative action, they form coalitions. Coalitions are a set of cliques formed around specific issues or events. They are less stable than cliques because the issues or events are temporary. A person may have membership in more than one clique or coalition.

The politics of an organization can be identified by how informal networks communicate and decisions occur. As a nurse manager, it is essential to understand the reasons behind the formation of cliques and coalitions. Efforts should be directed toward identifying the political behavior present in cliques and coalitions and choices made about whether to participate. Involvement in organizational politics is crucial when it promotes the goals of the organization. Therefore, attention should be paid to the kinds of interactions that occur in cliques and coalitions, remembering that all interaction has meaning and purpose. Managing the politics of cliques and coalitions requires an awareness of:

- **Power** unstable and not equally distributed (Cliques seek to maximize their own power base)
- **Decision making** occurs in a rational manner but through continued compromise, accommodation, and bargaining
- **Social gatherings** keys to holding the informal communication structures together (Who interacts with whom dur-

ing work, who helps out when, and whom do members view as the leader)

Nurse Manager As Group Leader and Politician

An effective nurse manager is a good politician. She or he is flexible and knows how to influence organizational environmental resources (personnel, money, time, and technology). Controlling and converting these resources into better patient care and increased productivity is functional politics. Functional politics is a form of self-interest behavior that promotes the goals of the organization. Through the use of politics, skills of influence, power (individual or collective), and authority the nurse manager develops a creative work environment that encourages the group to use their resources constructively. In addition to knowing what the group's resources are (members' talents, abilities, time, and money), the nurse manager knows how to interpret each member's behavior and approaches accordingly. This kind of political intervention provides vision of the group and reduces uncertainty about future allocation of scarce resources. The skillful manager strikes while the iron is hot—when the opportunity presents itself. Through effective communication the manager influences group members' behavior toward achievement of organizational goals.

Despite the growth of informal networks of cliques and coalitions, the nurse manager needs only to remember that members seek cliques and coalitions when there is a failure to recognize or respect members' needs to participate in formal organizational structures. Participation in organizational committees, interdisciplinary meetings, and staff in-service programs acknowledges members' abilities and talents. Nurse managers must be willing to share expertise and support their group as they attempt to influence organizational goals by asserting political muscle. If nurse managers use political skill within the organization, group members have the opportunity to learn these behaviors which can help them to gain broad-base support for their ideas, proposals, and programs.

As a role model, the nurse manager helps the group to understand the importance of organizational dynamics: its group interactions and relationships. Organizations are social systems and as such, have interdependent parts. A change in one part ripples out and influences other parts that in turn affect other parts (Tausley, 1976). The relationships among and between subsystems of the organization are constantly changing. All subsystems are not equal in their political behavior of power and influence. Some are more able to deal with critical sources of uncertainty about decisions and would appear more powerful. Power and status in the organization are not fixed and stable but constantly switching between groups and individuals. For instance, groups will act to decrease their internal dependence on others to limit uncertainty or lack of structure for the opportunity to grow and survive. The most important aspect of differentiation between groups is the development of particular norms and values to facilitate task accomplishment. The creation of these norms and values helps to create boundaries and an internal dynamics that adversely affects the ability to communicate between groups. The greater the differentiation between groups, the greater the distortion of communication and potential conflict. However, if groups are interdependent and must share scarce resources, then they must engage in joint problem solving and decision making.

To facilitate the sharing of scarce resources between groups, the nurse manager must have the ability to negotiate. Demonstrating control over critical resources builds the manager's stature and visibility in the organization. Specifically, the manager must use various sources of power to function effectively when interacting with cliques and coalitions. These sources of power include:

- **Coercive Power.** This power source is based on fear. Compliance is induced because failure to comply will result in punishment or penalties (French and Raven, 1959).
- **Connection Power.** A manager with connection power has bonds with influential and important people within and outside of an organization. By complying with the manager, followers believe that favor will be gained with the important people connected with their leader (Hersey, Blanchard, and Natemeyer, 1979).
- **Reward Power.** This is grounded on the belief of followers that the manager can provide rewards for them. Compliance with the manager's strategies results in gains such as increased pay and recognition (French and Raven, 1959).
- **Legitimate Power.** Based on a manager's position, followers believe that the manager has the right to influence them; their compliance follows. The higher one's position is, the more legitimate power one possesses (French and Raven, 1959).
- **Referent Power.** This source is based on the manager's personality trait; it is a part of one's personal power. A manager who is admired, liked, and identified with can induce compliance from followers (French and Raven, 1959).

- **Information Power.** Information power is based on possession of, or access to, information. This can influence people because of the belief that compliance will result in sharing of information; followers often have the need to be "in on things" (Raven and Kruglanski, 1977).
- **Expert Power.** Competence, knowledge, and skill are examples of expert power. Followers are influenced because their manager is seen as possessing the ability to facilitate accomplishment of their goals and objectives (French and Raven, 1959).

Possessing a solid power base is crucial, and using the appropriate source of power at any given time is essential. As nurse manager, you must be willing to reward and punish when needed, share expertise, issue directives, follow up on compliance, and attempt to influence as the occasion arises. Managers are expected to assess what source of power can best improve work performance and must demonstrate the managerial competence to produce desired results. Producing desired results often leads to conflict. Conflict is inevitable when trying to influence others to improve their productivity.

CONFLICT IN THE NURSING ORGANIZATION

Nurse managers may have different opinions as to the needs and methods of accomplishing desired results than those of group members. It is a natural consequence of self-interest behavior. Deutsch (1973) defines conflict as a clash or struggle that occurs when one's feelings, thoughts, desires, and behavior are threatened. This struggle can be within an individual or within a group. Conflict is a learned behavior arising from within, between, and among individuals because of differences in facts, views, goals, and authority. Conflict is described as an expressed struggle between at least two interdependent parties, who perceive incompatible goals, scarce rewards, and interference from the other party in achieving their goals. They are in a position of opposition in conjunction with cooperation (Deutsch, p. 9).

Conflict is inevitable in the nursing organization. It can be classified as vertical or horizontal (Marriner, 1979). Vertical conflict involves differences between superiors and subordinates or between labor and management. It results from poor communication and a lack of shared perceptions regarding expectations of appropriate behavior for one's role and that of others (La Monica, 1983, p. 210). Horizontal conflict arises from line-staff conflict and usually involves areas of authority, expertise, and practice. Vertical and horizontal conflict can be moderated, though never completely eliminated from organizational life.

In every situation there are three levels of conflict: (1) *perceived conflict*, the realization that conditions exist between groups or within self that can cause conflict; (2) *felt conflict*, the conflict brings out feelings of threat, hostility, fear, or mistrust between groups; (3) *expressed conflict*, the conflict takes the form of active or passive interference by at least one group with another in debate, assertion, competition, or problem-solving.

CONFLICT MANAGEMENT AND RESOLUTION

Managing conflict is not an easy task for any manager. The ideal way of handling conflict is to lessen the perceptual differences that exist. This way the nurse manager can deal with and resolve conflict that may affect the performance, productivity, and communication among and between group members. Deutsch (1973) suggests three possible solutions of conflict:

1. The win/lose resolution uses various methods by a group or individual to obtain its goals and deliberately attempts to frustrate the other group or individual. Win/lose is a frequent resolution to conflict but not a desirable one in that the losing party is left with feelings of frustration and anger that can lead to renewed conflict.
2. The lose/lose resolution is when each group gives up some desired goals through compromise and neither group gets all. This is an undesired resolution since each group has a feeling of defeat as a result of a lose/lose compromise.
3. The win/win resolution is the ideal resolution for conflict. Both groups identify solutions that allow them each to achieve their goals; both feel that they have created a resolution that they can live with.

To lessen the probability of a continuation of conflict in the future, the win/win resolution offers the following three approaches to manage conflict: structural, process, and mixed (Nadler, Hackman, and Lawler, 1979).

The structural approach requires the use of devices such as setting of common goals, reward systems, regrouping, and separation of groups to resolve conflict. In setting of common goals, there is a creation of a superordinate goal. This superordinate goal is something that the group desires to achieve beyond the conflict.

In the structural approach, the reward system acknowledges both groups for reaching their desired goals and avoids penalizing one group at the expense of another. Regrouping or joining conflicting groups together into a larger unit with a common goal helps to reduce conflict. Last, the physical or structural separation of interdependent groups into different units or areas where they are no longer interdependent on each other can be used if all else fails.

The second approach for a win/win resolution is the process approach that requires the intervention of a skilled third party in the conflict episode. The third party must possess experience in negotiation, conflict resolution, or counseling. The process approach consists of three methods: de-escalation, confrontation, and collaboration. In de-escalation, one party stops reacting to the other party in a hostile way. This tends to elicit similar behavior from the conflicting party. The second process approach, originated by Becklar (1969), is confrontation. This is also accomplished with a skilled third-party mediator. Confrontation allows later parties to vent their grievances and seek a solution to the conflict. The third process approach is collaboration, whereby both parties work together to try to resolve their conflicts.

The third approach uses mixed solutions in win/win resolution. Here, the structural and process approaches are combined. In the mixed approach, the organization will structurally develop rules for conflict resolution. Many organizations have developed these rules through labor contracts. An example of this is the grievance procedure, whereby an employee can bring perceived problems to the attention of management. A second structural approach in the mixed mode is the *liaison role*, where a third party is built into the organizational structure and that third party is available to aid in the win/win conflict resolution. An example of someone in the liaison role would be a grievance officer, a patient advocate, or an ombudsman.

Another type of mixed resolution is the task force or team approach that creates teams made up of group members that span the normal boundaries of groups that might tend to have conflict. At the head of the team would be someone acting as coordinator or investigator. For example, in the event of conflict between medical and nursing disciplines an interdisciplinary team would be devised to deal with resolution of conflict, with a neutral coordinator to help mediate the conflict.

The mixed approach to conflict resolution offers the best approach in resolving organizational conflict because conflict is so inherent in organizations that it tends to be better to build in the processes for resolution of the conflict rather than to try and resolve each conflict with a new set of structures or processes as they arise. Examples of a mixed approach to conflict resolution include an organization's grievance procedures and rules of arbitration.

The ability to successfully manage conflict is an important skill for the nurse manager in today's nursing organization. Knowledge of the dynamics of conflict processes is essential, if the nurse manager is to become sensitive to events that trigger the conflict cycle. In addition, knowledge about barriers that prevent individuals and/or groups from initiating or reacting to conflict behavior is also necessary. Knowing how to manage conflict helps the nurse manager to minimize the cost and increase the benefits to the group and overall organization's productivity and goals.

LABOR RELATIONS: A MEANS OF CONFLICT RESOLUTION IN NURSING ORGANIZATIONS

Since the passage of the amendments of the National Labor Relations Act of 1974, professional nurses perceive collective bargaining as a viable alternative for resolving conflict between themselves and management. Prior to 1974, not-for-profit hospitals were excluded from all provisions of the National Labor Relations Act (see Table 4–1, which reviews the history of Labor Relations Law). The amendment removed the not-for-profit hospital exemption, thus allowing hospital employees right of protection to engage in union activity without interference and/or reprisal by their employers (see Table 4–2, the Taft–Hartley Amendments). The purpose of collective bargaining in health care organizations is to secure for nurses reasonable and satisfactory conditions of employment, which, in turn, will enable the public to secure top quality nursing service in sufficient quantity (Flanagan, 1976). Collective bargaining is the process by which unions

TABLE 4–1. A HISTORICAL REVIEW OF LABOR RELATIONS LAW

1935	Passage of the National Labor Relations Act (the Wagner Act). Conferred the right upon private sector employees to engage in union activity.
1947	Taft–Hartley Amendments of the National Labor Relations Act. Excluded from its coverage employees of not-for-profit hospitals and placed restraints of unfair labor practices on unions.
1974	Amendments to Taft–Hartley. Removed the exemption of not-for-profit hospitals.

TABLE 4–2. THE 1974 TAFT–HARTLEY AMENDMENTS

Defined the term health care institution to include any hospital, convalescent hospital, health maintenance organization, nursing home, extended care facility, or any other institution that cares for the sick, infirm, or aged.

Set a 90-day notice period for negotiations or collective bargaining contracts. This 90-day notice by either the employer or labor organization is required for renewals or modifications of contracts, rather than the 60-day notice required for all other industries covered by the National Labor Relations Act.

Required that the Federal Mediation and Conciliation Service is notified 60 days before the termination of an existing contract, as opposed to the 30-day notification required for other industries.

Required labor organizations to participate in the mediation process in both renewal and initial contract situations.

Required written notices by the labor organizations to the health care institution and the Federal Mediation and Conciliation Service 10 days before engaging in any picketing, strike, or other concerted refusal to work. There are no strike or picketing notice provisions in the act for other industries.

Before the expiration of the notification periods on renewal and initial contracts, and the discretion of the director of the Federal Mediation and Conciliation Service, an impartial board of inquiry could be established to investigate any labor–management dispute and make a written report on its findings. This process judges whether an actual or a threatened work stoppage could substantially interrupt the delivery of health care to the community involved. There is no provision for other industries covered under the act.

An employee of a health care institution who is a member of a recognized religion, body, or sect that historically held conscientious objections to participation in or support of labor organizations will not be required to join or financially support such an organization as a condition of employment. This position applies to health care institutions only as defined within the act.

The 1975 amendments to the National Labor Relations Act preempt all state labor laws previously applicable to nongovernmental hospitals. Also, the amendments apply to health care institutions previously covered by the act (such as proprietary hosptials and nursing homes) as well as to all those institutions brought under federal law by the amendments to the act.

After McConnell, C. The effective health care supervisor. Rockville, Md.: Aspen, 1982.

share in the management decisions involving the terms of employment and the price of labor (Flanagan, 1976).

When limited autonomy, lack of communication with management, and exclusion from decision making in nursing practices are present, the potential for conflict arises. These sources of dissatisfaction act as significant reasons why nurses join unions. The struggle for control over practice, job satisfaction, and economic security are paramount to professional employment. Nurses who engage in collective bargaining believe it to be the only solution to the labor–management power struggle. The vulnerability of union organizing in any health care organization can originate from any of the following labor–management conflicts (McConnell, 1984).

Input into Organizational Decision Making
- Employees feel that they have no input into the decisions affecting their work
- Employees receive no management response to their suggestions, problems, and questions

Problem-Solving Process
- There is no formal, consistent, multistep problem or grievance resolution procedure
- Discipline is not applied fairly, uniformly, and consistently
- Disciplinary actions are taken without extending to employees a reasonable opportunity to correct their behavior

Quality of Supervision
- Insufficient attention is given to placing managers out of consideration for communications skills, leadership, and problem-solving abilities
- Top management fails to act on apparent supervisory weaknesses: discrimination, harassment, favoritism, neglect, and so on
- No effort is made to stimulate upward communication, and few channels are open to employees

Organizational Stability and Job Security
- There are frequent shifts in workload and work distribution
- There is a history of instability, leading the employees to anticipate periodic layoffs
- Surprise changes occur in job structure and assignments
- New methods and new equipment are introduced without advance notice

Compensation and Benefits
- Pay rates are not comparable with other health care organizations
- There is no reflection on individual performance in the granting of raises
- There are internal inequities in pay
- Employees do not understand how their pay is determined

- There is no job evaluation program or other systematic approach to grading jobs and thus for setting rates of pay

Working Conditions
- Hazardous or unpleasant tasks or physical areas are not addressed and controlled
- There is no formal safety program and no apparent attention given to employee safety
- There is widespread dissatisfaction with physical facilities and employee services (cafeteria service, parking, workplace decor, etc.)

If properly explored by management and labor relations, the above-named conflict situations would be avoided, thus preventing unionization from occurring. However, it requires that management be willing to engage in open dialogue with labor, be proactive rather than reactive to problems, and be willing to listen without making promises or commitments that will not be implemented. Organizations that foster the manager–employee relationship through clever and simple communication structures reduce internal conflicts. If the communication becomes unclear and distorted between the manager and the employee, distance or indifference builds and conflict proliferates. It follows then that an unresolved conflict between labor and management is a fertile ground for union-organizing activity. Thus, a key responsibility that a nurse manager has is to maintain a communicating relationship in the manager–employee relationship. Communication flows easily from one person to another. Here the nurse manager strives to keep the communication channel open with a full exchange of information. This effort helps to maintain awareness of possible problems and reduce conflicts.

The Nurse Manager's Role in Collective Bargaining

When organizational communication becomes ineffective and collective bargaining ensues, it places tremendous responsibilities on the nurse manager. He or she may not have direct involvement in the collective bargaining process but will have to implement the outcomes of contract negotiations. The nurse manager must learn the contract thoroughly—learn what it means inside out. Unionization creates a need for increased knowledge and skills in areas of labor relations, such as grievance proceedings, selection of personnel, performance appraisals, and effective discipline. The primary responsibility of the nurse manager will be to develop a model of labor relations that will benefit not only the professional employee and management, but the patient, as well. A skillful manager blends the provisions of the labor contract into the department's goals, thus directing energy away from ongoing conflicts between management and employees. All interactions between the manager and the employee are open and honest, regardless of what the contract contains. It is essential to remember that the employees work for the organization, not for the union. It is also important for the nurse manager to realize that she or he is a member of the management team whom the employees know best—you are the manager that supervises the people who provide the hands-on care. The employees see the nurse manager as a representative of all management and the organization. Therefore, sound labor relations skills, such as a caring and concerned attitude toward employees, effective communications, and negotiation are reflective of the entire management team and organization.

Collective bargaining in a health care organization is sometimes perceived as a deficit by management. This is not necessarily true. Collective bargaining in service professions is a current reality. It exists because unions strive to improve the working conditions and economic status of their members; because of the occupational sexism experienced by nurses—low pay, low status for women's work. Collective bargaining offers a power base to nurses that can protect their personal and professional welfare. Once collective bargaining is established within the organization, the object of management should be to smooth relationships and work within the existing structure of the contract.

REFERENCES AND BIBLIOGRAPHY

Becklar, R. *Organizational development: Strategies and models.* Reading, Mass.: Addison-Wesley, 1969.

Bennis, W, & Nanus, B. *Leaders.* New York: Harper & Row, Pub., 1985.

Cartwright, D., & Zander, A. *A group dynamics: Research and theory.* New York: Harper & Row, Pub., 1968.

Collins, B.E., & Guetzkow, H.A. *A social psychology of group process for decision-making.* New York: Wiley, 1964.

Deutsch, M. *The resolution of conflict: Constructive and destructive processes.* New Haven: Yale University Press, 1973.

Flanagan, L. *One strong voice: The story of the American Nurses' Association.* Kansas City: American Nurses' Association, 1976.

French, J., & Raven, B. The bases of social power. In D. Cartwright (Ed.). *Studies in Social Power.* Ann Arbor: University of Michigan, 1959.

Hersey, P., & Blanchard, K. *Management of organizational behavior: Utilizing human resources* (3rd ed.). Englewood Cliffs, N.J.: Prentice Hall, 1977.

Hersey, P., Blanchard, K., & Natemeyer, W. *Situational leadership, perception, and impact of power.* La Jolla, Calif.: Learning Resources, 1979.

La Monica, E. *Nursing leadership and management.* Monterey, Calif.: Wadsworth Health Science, 1983.

Marriner, A. Conflict theory. *Supervisor Nurse*, 1979, 46, 52–54.

McConnell, C. *Managing the health care professional.* Rockville, Md.: Aspen, 1984.

Nadler, D., Hackman, J.R., & Lawler, E. *Managing organizational behavior.* Boston: Little, Brown, 1979.

Peters, T., & Waterman, R. *In search of excellence.* New York: Harper & Row, pub., 1982.

Raven, B., & Kruglanski, A. Conflict and power. in P. Shingle (Ed.). *The structure of conflict.* New York: Academia Press, 1970.

Robbins, S. The administrative press. Englewood Cliffs, N.J.: Prentice Hall, 1976.

Tausley, C. Theories of organization. In W. Nord (Ed.). *Concepts and controversy in organizational behavior* (2nd ed.). Santa Monica, Calif.: Good Year, 1976.

Vroom, V., & Yetton, P. *Leadership and decision-making.* Pittsburgh: University of Pittsburgh Press, 1973.

CHAPTER 5

Leadership in the Nursing Organization

We have examined thus far the nursing organization as an open system; the role of the nurse manager; the motivation of the individual in the nursing organization; and the functioning of groups in the nursing organization. We come then to an examination of leadership in the nursing organization. Much has been written about leadership in nursing and most nurse managers will probably have had at least one course in nursing leadership sometime in their career. Why then another discussion of leadership? Because *leadership* has often been confused with *management* in nursing literature. A review of classical leadership theory lays a foundation that helps illuminate some newer theories of leadership. Business psychologist Abraham Zaleznick stated, "Managers prefer working with people; leaders stir emotion" (1977, p. 72). James McGregor Burns, in his classic book, *Leadership*, defined two types of leaders: the *transactional leader* and the *transformational leader*. Burns states:

> The relations of most leaders and followers are transactional—leaders approach followers with an eye to exchanging one thing for another: jobs for votes, or subsidies for campaign contributions. Such transactions compromise the bulk of the relationships among leaders and followers, especially in groups, legislatures, and parties. (1978, p.4)

The *transactional leader* correlates with the concept of a manager put forth by Zalesznick as one who enjoys working with people and has some administration skills. *Transforming leaders,* on the other hand, are visionaries—those who can stir emotion. Can we influence leadership behavior? Can we develop a strong leadership base in our nursing organizations? A close examination of the function of leadership in the organization can help us to answer these questions.

If we examine the structure of organizations, we realize that these structures are imperfect and that gaps exist in the organizational structure. These gaps may be thought of as *boundaries* and leadership within the organization can be conceptualized as a *boundary-spanning function*. That is, leaders bridge gaps between the external environment and the internal environment of the organization. This allows followers to perform their tasks within the organization. The bigger the gap, the more leeway there is for acts of leadership. Because the nursing organization is an open system, constantly interacting with its environment and receiving feedback about its output, change is constant. Certain changes are handled routinely. For example, fluctuations in patient census and acuity, which influence staffing and scheduling patterns, become a routine part of the input that is manipulated to have a smoothly functioning organization. However, major changes and fluctuations in the environment may require adustments beyond the usual routine changes. It is in times of major change that the organization requires true leadership and not merely management.

Katz and Kahn describe three types of leadership behavior in organizations depending on the level in the organization at which the leader functions.

1. *Top echelon.* Introduction of structural change or policy formulation. This is the most challenging kind of leadership, but not the most frequent.
2. *Middle management.* Interpolation of existing structure, i.e., piecing out the incompleteness in existing structures and improvising within the limits of the existing structure.
3. *First line supervisory level.* Using existing formal structures for maintenance of organizational operations. Figure 5–1 illustrates Katz and Kahn's conception of the leadership process in organizations and the cognitive affective abilities and skills needed by leaders at the various levels of the organization. (1978, pp. 536–539)

It is Katz and Kahn's premise that leadership skills required at one level of the organization may not be functional at another level. Their belief is that different cognitive and affective skills are necessary, depending on the level of leadership in the organization. This concept of leadership in organizations leaves room

Type of Leadership Process	Typical Organizational Level	Abilities and Skills	
		Cognitive	Affective
Origination: change, creation, and elimination of structure	Top echelons	System perspective	Charisma
Interpolation: supplementing and piecing out of structure	Intermediate levels: pivotal roles	Subsystem perspective: two-way orientation	Integration of primary and secondary relations human relations skills
Administration: use of existing structure	Lower levels	Technical knowledge and understanding of system of rules	Concern with equity in use of rewards and sanctions

Figure 5–1. Leadership patterns, their locus in the organization, and their skill requirements. *(From Katz and Kahn. Social Psychology of Organizations, Wiley, 1978. Reprinted with permission.)*

for different types of leadership within the nursing organization. There may be talented leaders at various levels of the organization with skills and abilities that allow their leadership to flourish at that level.

Some may move up through the various echelons of the nursing organization because they possess the abilities and skills, on cognitive and affective levels, which are necessary for the leadership functions at a higher level. It behooves the managers in the nursing organization to be aware of the skills and abilities needed by nursing leaders and managers from first line supervisors through to the chief executive officers of nursing. By assessing the skills and abilities of potential leaders, we can foster their growth and development. A systematic look at the development of leadership theory can give us some insights into how to initiate leadership development in our organizations.

CLASSICAL LEADERSHIP THEORIES

The Ohio State leadership studies form the basis for much of the leadership theory that followed these studies of the 1940s. The Ohio State research was based on measuring two basic dimensions of leadership behavior:

- *Initiating structure*, which is the relationship between superiors and subordinates that establishes defined patterns of organization, communication, and procedure
- *Consideration*, which is behavior that indicates friendship, trust, warmth, interest, and respect

A questionnaire known as the Leadership Behavior Questionnaire (LBDQ) results in a four-quadrant design that rates leaders high or low on the two dimensions of initiating structure and consideration.

Figure 5–2 illustrates the four quadrants formed by using the LBDQ dimensions. The Ohio State studies rated quadrant I as the most effective leadership category, with some effectiveness also occurring in Quadrants II and IV. It found the least effective leaders falling into Quadrant III. The Ohio State studies did not conclusively determine one best form of leadership behavior. The results of the study gave rise to new research questions.

Fiedler's Contingency Model

The work of Fiedler built on the Ohio State studies and added a new dimension to the study of leadership behavior. Fiedler added the dimension of the *situation* to the two factors of initiating

Quadrant II	Quandrant I
Low consideration	High consideration
High initiating	High initiating
structure	structure
Quandrant III	Quandrant IV
Low consideration	High consideration
Low initiating	Low initiating
structure	structure

Figure 5–2. The LBDQ leadership behavior quadrants.

structure and consideration. Fiedler differentiated between *leadership behavior* and *leadership style*, defining leadership behavior as that specific behavior used while directing and controlling the work of a unit. Leadership style is defined as the underlying attitudes toward people, which motivate the leader's behavior i.e., her or his personality. The underlying assumption of Fiedler's work is that in different situations, different leadership behaviors are required. Fiedler defined three factors that influence the favorableness of the situation for the leader (1967).

1. Position power. The formal power of the leader's position in the organization.
2. Task structure. How clearly a task is defined by the leader and by the organization. The more structured the task, the more favorable the situation for the leader.
3. Leader–member relations. The extent to which the leader is respected and accepted by his or her followers. This is in part determined by the personality and behavior of the leader. Table 5–1 illustrates the classification of leadership

TABLE 5–1. FAVORABLENESS OF THE SITUATION AS A FACTOR IN LEADER EFFECTIVENESS

Degree of Favorableness of the Situation for the Leader	Task Structure	Position Power of Leader	Leader– Member Relations
Favorable	Structured	High	Good
	Structured	Low	Good
	Unstructured	High	Good
Moderately favorable	Unstructured	Low	Good
	Structured	High	Poor
	Structured	Low	Poor
	Unstructured	High	Poor
Unfavorable	Unstructured	Low	Poor

After Fiedler 1967.

situations according to their degree of favorableness for the leader, taking into consideration the factors of position power, task, structure, and leader–member relations.

The concept of favorableness of a given situation to various leadership styles was further developed in the work of Hersey and Blanchard.

The Situational Theory of Leadership

Hersey and Blanchard (1977) took Fiedler's contingency concept further and defined favorableness in terms of the *maturity of the group* with which the leader is working. Group maturity is defined as the degree to which the group is familiar with the task at hand. It does not have to do with the length of time a person is employed in the organization and certainly not with the age or professional experience of the employee.

A leader may have an experienced group of workers who are confronted with a new task to perform. That group would be assessed as immature regarding the performance of that particular task. For example, an experienced group of head nurses who were required to do their own budgeting for the first time would be regarded as immature in that task, and would, therefore, require a more directive leadership approach for a time.

The Hersey–Blanchard situational leadership theory uses the maturity of the group and the elements of task and relationship that parallel the quadrants of the Ohio State leadership studies. In essence, the situational theory contends that working with people who are low in maturity in terms of accomplishing a specific task requires a high task–low relationship style. As the group matures in its ability to accomplish a task, the leadership style can become one of high relationship and low task orientation. In the Hersey–Blanchard model, the most mature groups require the least leader direction, either in relationship or task. The situational theory defines four leadership styles: *S1 telling* is characterized by high task orientation and low interpersonal orientation that is not related to the task. *S2 behavior* is high in task and high in relationship and is referred to as *selling style* because the leader attempts a two-way communication and socioemotional support to get the folowers to "buy into" the decisions that have to be made.

S3 is termed the *participating style* and is the high relationship, low task behavior needed for a group that is familiar with the task and needs more personal reinforcement. *S4* is labeled the *delegating style* because the leader allows followers who are very mature in their task to, in effect, run their own show (Hersey and Blanchard, 1977). The situational leadership theory can be seen to combine the elements of the Ohio State studies, which identified task and consideration as the primary elements of leadership style, and the contingency of the situation, introduced by Fiedler's research.

The Blake and Mouton Managerial Grid

The Blake and Mouton managerial grid presents another model of leadership behavior that is based on the concepts of relationships with people, and concern for productivity, or the basic elements of initiating structure and consideration. The grid has two axes that go from 0 to 9 with a potential of 81 points, and can identify very specific leadership behaviors. However, Blake and Mouton identified *five basic leadership styles* that characterize most leadership (Blake and Mouton, 1964). The 1–1 style of impoverished leadership can be equated with quadrant III of the Ohio State grid; that is a leader low in consideration and low in initiating structure or, as defined by Blake and Mouton, low in concern for people and low in concern for production.

Blake and Mouton's ideal leader is the 9–9, which could be equated to quadrant I of the Ohio State grid. The 9–9 leader demonstrates a high concern for people as well as a high concern for productivity. The managerial grid indicates that most leaders fall somewhere short of the 9–9 style and that many will fall into the 5–5 category of balanced leadership. The difference between 5–5 leadership and 9–9 leadership may be what Burns is describing as the difference between the transactional leader and the transforming leader.

NEW APPROACHES TO LEADERSHIP DEVELOPMENT

It can be seen that most of the classical leadership theories have focused on the elements of a manager's orientation to either the task or the people in the situation. There is great similarity between the various theories and their dependence on the basic two elements of task and people, or concern for productivity and concern for human resources. Newer work on leadership has led to the concept of leadership as a much more complex phenomenon that cannot easily be explained on a two-dimensional theory or even by situational or contingency theories of leadership. Although much has been written about leadership in nursing, there is a dearth of research about leadership characteristics of nurse managers in particular. Research regarding nurses and leadership styles or characteristics has been traditionally focused on nurses in positions of deans of schools of nursing or centered on personality characteristics of staff nurses.

Such studies use the LBDQ, which measures the two dimensions of concern for people and concern for task, or focus on the personality characteristics of nurses in leadership positions. There is little normative data about leadership characteristics of nurses in middle management positions or about factors that can influence the leadership styles and characteristics of these nurse managers. Effective management development programs that will increase nurse manager's ability to lead are dependent on some understanding of the leadership characteristics of nurse managers as a group. Some light may be shed on the leadership characteristics of nurse managers by a research study conducted by the author that examines leadership characteristics of nurse managers before and after completion of a master's degree program in nurse management.

The study shows that *dependency* as a dominant characteristic is significantly reduced after completion of a master's degree program. It further shows an increase in scores in such positive leadership characteristics as humanistic/helpful and achievement (see Appendix B for a detailed description of the study).

Pressure for change in our health care system and in our nursing organizations will intensify, not diminish, in the coming years. The pressure for change from the environment requires nursing organizations to respond with new and dynamic leadership at every level of the organization. We will need leadership that is *transformational*, rather than *transactional*, to cope with future changes.

ASPIRING TO TRANSFORMATIONAL LEADERSHIP

James McGregor Burns, in his Pulitzer Prize wininng book *Leadership* (1978), identifed two leadership types: the *transactional* and the *transformational*. His work has cast a new meaning on the word *leadership* and the study of leadership.

Transactional Leadership

The *transactional* type of leadership is the most common one found in organizations. Transactional leaders approach followers with an eye to exchanging one thing for another; promotions for support of policies; favored consideration for loyalty. The concept is one of "one hand washes the other." Transactional leaders tend to move organizations along historical tracks, making only minor adjustments to the organization's mission, structure, and human resource management. Most leadership in organizations today is transactional and there is nothing basically wrong with that. Transactional leadership does serve to keep organizations on track in the routine functions. However, in times of change something more is required.

Transforming leadership is much more complex and more potent. "The transforming leader recognizes and exploits an existing need or demand of potential followers. Transforming leadership is a relationship of mutual stimulation and elevation that converts followers into leaders" (Burns, 1978, p. 4). The transforming leader is able to develop a *new vision* of the organization and to communicate that vision to others. This kind of leader has the ability to get others to commit themselves to this new vision. How are transforming leaders able to do this?

Through the revamping of its *technical, political,* and *cultural* systems, an organization can be led to revitalization. In the coming decades of increased information, competition, and technological advances, there will be continuing signs that change is indicated and needed in the nursing organization. The signs may be called *trigger events* in the organization's environment. These so-called trigger events indicate when change is needed, and are readily sensed by transformational leaders (Tichy and Ulrich, 1984). We do not have to look far to find trigger events in today's health care industry. The advent of prospective payment systems, high technology in medicine and nursing, computerization in health care agencies, are all trigger events that have indicated the need for change within the nursing organization. We must assume, however, that leaders and organizations that respond to trigger events by initiating change generate mixed feelings and various kinds of resistance to that very change. The forces of resistance to change are generated in three interrelated systems: *technical system resistance, political systems resistance,* and *cultural systems resistance.*

Technical System Resistance. Habit and inertia are two major factors in technical system resistance. Individuals in organizations do things in a certain way. Changing the way things are done can meet with great resistance. The change over from the usual system of patient record keeping to a hospital information system that is computerized can cause fear and great inertia and resistance on the part of the staff, for example. We must also realize that organizational resources are heavily committed to the

old technical systems, or ways of doing things, within an organization. When change is introduced we are also talking about
committing additional resources, and discarding technical systems that may have been used in the old way of doing things,
thus increasing resistance on technical grounds.

Political Systems Resistance. Powerful coalitions exist within
any organization. Conflict can arise between the old guard and
the new guard. The limitation of resources can force decisions
regarding the decrease in size of certain units in an organization
and the transfer or termination of certain workers. These kinds
of changes can initiate political resistance. Also, there may be
present what Tichy and Ulrich describe as "the quality of in-
dictment," which refers to the leader who was party to creating
the problems that exist in the organization. Identifying problems
that require organizational change may have a quality of indict-
ment of the leader about it. It is sometimes easier for new leaders
to come into an organization and initiate change because they do
not have to indict themselves everytime they indicate something
is wrong with the organization. Indeed, people often expect new
leaders to initiate change.

Cultural Systems Resistance. Resistance within the culture of
the organization may be the most important consideration of all.
People find security based on past experience. More importantly,
people in organizations may have *cultural filters* that keep them
from being able to conceive or envision another way of doing
things. An outsider or perhaps some deviant in the organization
may be able to perceive a way of change that most in the organization cannot. In many organizations that require a great deal
of conformity, such as health care organizations and hospitals,
there may be the lack of a climate for change. When a great deal
of conformity is required in an organization, entrepreneurship
and change are not encouraged, and therefore, it may be difficult
to institute change in these organizations.

Leaders must be aware of the three resistances to change
in organizations. The difference between transactional leadership
and transformational leadership is in meeting these forces of resistance. The transactional leader is not able to challenge these
resistances adequately, and therefore, instead of change and
growth, we may find organizational decline. The transformational
leader, on the other hand, is able to *create a vision* of the desired
state of the new organization. This vision is congruent with the
leader's and the organization's philosophy and style. There are

many different ways to achieve desired change; however, creating a vision is essential.

Creating a Vision

In some organizations creating and communicating a vision may be done through a great deal of committee work and staff work in decision making. In other organizations it may be done by an intuitive, directive leader who depends on charisma to create a vision for the organization. In addition to the creation of the vision, the transforming leader must be able to mobilize a critical mass of the organization to accept this vision and to make it happen. A transforming leader must have *commitment* from the members of the organization—*the leader cannot make change happen alone.*

From mobilization and commitment to changing the technical, political, and cultural systems of the organization grow the institutionalization of change. The changes created must become solidly entrenched in the organization. One way this can be done is through the alteration of communication and decision-making processes. Another and crucial way that the transforming leader reinforces and institutionalizes change is by reinforcing the new *organizational culture*. Cultural systems in organizations do not just occur randomly; they occur because leaders spend time on, and reward some behaviors and practices more than others. Those behaviors that are rewarded become the valued norms of the organization. Leaders can then shape new cultures by carefully monitoring where and how they spend their time and by encouraging and rewarding the employee behaviors that they value. Transforming leaders are aware that where and how their time is spent helps to shape the culture, beliefs, and norms of the organization.

If a middle manager spends a great deal of time on the quality assurance function, for instance, the staff will respond by also valuing the procedures involved in collecting data for quality assurance. If, on the other hand, a middle manager values excellent communications with staff and is known to frequently tour subunits to assess potential problems, then open communication will be perceived as valued in the organization and will set the behavioral norms. Culture provides an organization's members with a *way of understanding symbols* and *events*. It provides meaning to those who function within the organization.

What qualities does the transformational leader need to possess to transform the technical, political, and cultural resistances in the organization? First, we must accept the fact that not everyone can be a transformational leader. There is always a need for transactional leadership, which maintains organizations by carrying out day-to-day tasks. When transformational leaders evolve, they have a deep understanding, whether it be intuitive or learned, of organizations, their functioning, and their place in society. "Thus, as a start, transformational leaders need to understand concepts of equity, power, freedom, and the dynamics of decision-making" (Tichy and Ulrich, 1984, p. 67). The transforming leader knows when to react to a trigger event and when to seize the opportunity.

This requires more than being in the right place at the right time; it is really superb timing. Finally, the transforming leader needs to know how to articulate the new vision, values, and norms and how to use various avenues to support the new culture of the organization. This can be done in a variety of ways such as *role modeling, symbolic acts of reward* for desired behaviors, *creation of rituals* within the organization, *revamping of human resource systems,* and *changing the management processes within the organization.* Each leader will find the avenues that are most compatible with her or his leadership style and organization. There is no formula for beginning to change an organization through transformational leadership. There are numerous ways to approach change, but based on the premise that the pressure for change in nursing and health care delivery will intensify, we must have transformational leaders for the future. We must nurture, encourage, and support the growth of transformational leaders in nursing. Based on the author's research into the leadership characteristics of nurse managers, graduate preparation can make a significant difference in the development of strong leadership qualities.

To exert influence as leaders and to aspire to transformational leadership, we must ask ourselves some crucial questions (Burns, 1978).

1. What are our personal goals? What are the career goals of the person who aspires to or attains a leadership position? We must decide whether we are really trying to lead anyone but ourselves and what part of ourselves and for what purpose. Many who attain leadership positions do so merely to advance their own careers. Career advancement is a legitimate reason for aspiring to leadership positions; however, potential leaders must be aware of when their own personal goals are the driving force behind their reach for leadership positions.

2. Whom are we seeking to lead? No one can be a leader without followers. Burns has emphasized the synergistic mutuality between leader and follower that is necessary for true transforming leadership. The transforming leader must define who the followers are in terms of their mutuality and future motives as well as in terms of what resistances might be met by the leader in trying to institute change.

3. Where are we seeking to go? The true transforming leaders have a vision of a future desired state for the organization. They do not initiate change for change's sake. They understand what they would like the organization to look like and they are able to translate this vision into institutional change. A true transforming leader is one who is able to realize a goal of *real and intended change*.

A word must be said here about the difference between leadership and power. Much has been written about the attainment of power in nursing, and the need for nurses to have power. There is a difference between true leadership and mere power.

> Leadership, unlike naked power wielding, is thus inseparable from followers' needs and goals. The essence of the leader–follower relation is the interaction of persons with different levels of motivations and of power potential, including skill, in pursuit of a common or at least a joint purpose. Naked power wielding can be neither transactional nor transforming; *only leadership can be*. (Burns, 1978, pp. 19–20)

REFERENCES

Blake R., & Mouton, J. *The managerial grid*, Houston, Tx.: Gulf Publishing, 1964.

Brooten, D. *Managerial leadership in nursing*. Philadelphia: Lippincott, 1984.

Burns, J.McG. *Leadership*. New York: Harper & Row, Pub., 1978.

Fiedler, F. *A theory of leadership effectiveness*. New York: McGraw-Hill, 1967.

Hemphill, J., & Coons, A. *Leader behavior description*. Columbus, Oh.: Personal Research Board, Ohio State University, 1950.

Hersey, P., & Blanchard, K. *Management of organizational behavior: Utilizing human resources* (3rd ed.). Englewood Cliffs, N.J.: Prentice Hall, 1977.

Kantor, R.H. *The charge masters*. New York: Simon & Schuster, 1983.

Katz, D. & Kahn, R. *The social psychology of organizations*. New York: Wiley, 1978.

Kirsch, J. *Leadership characteristics of nurse managers* (Research presentation). NYSNA, October, 1985.

Lafferty, C. *Level I: Life styles inventory.* Plymouth, Mich.: Human Synergistics, 1982.

Tappen, R.M. *Nursing leadership: Concepts and practice.* Philadelphia: F.A. Davis Company, 1983.

Tichy, N., & Ulrich, D. The leadership challenge—A call for the transformational leader. *Sloan Management Review*, 1984, *26*(1), 59–68.

Zaleznick, A. Managers and leaders: Are they different. *Harvard Business Review*, May-June, 1977, 72–84.

CHAPTER 6

Decision Making in the Nursing Organization

Nursing managers make decisions as a large part of their work. Decisions must be made about the allocation of human and fiscal resources within the nursing organization. Decisions are made that initiate change and decisions are made about the many issues that arise daily in organizations and require action. Some decisions are made routinely, following set guidelines or policies. Some are made almost by reflex, within seconds. Others must be pondered and indeed may be pondered for days or weeks. Many important policy-level decisions are made by groups of people within the organization and may be made after deliberative study over a fairly long period of time. Regardless of how decisions are made in organizations, individuals are the key to decision making. Therefore, it behooves us to look at the individual and the various types of fallibility in the decision-making process to which human beings fall heir. This chapter explores some of the classic decision-making models and some newer concepts about the process of decision making in organizations.

THE COGNITIVE MODEL OF DECISION MAKING

The cognitive model of decision making is based on the notion of rational choice. This is the classical model of problem solving, which has its origins in the work of Dewey (1910) and the four stages of problem solution. The four stages of decision making of the classical model are familiar to nurses who have found them

93

in other guises such as the nursing process. The classical four steps are:

1. *Defining the problem.* Clarifying exactly what the problem is, is the crucial first step in the decision-making process. We can include in this first stage the gathering of information or the collection of data about the problem.
2. *Generating alternative solutions.* This stage involves the generation of alternative solutions to the problem and the examination of these alternatives in terms of their feasibility.
3. *Evaluation of the consequences.* This step looks at and considers the consequences of various alternative solutions and tries to anticipate the probability of various outcomes if a given solution is chosen.
4. *Implementation of a solution.* Once one of the alternative solutions to a problem is chosen, it must be implemented. Decisions about how to implement a solution or an alternative may be a process in decision making in itself.

These four steps may vary slightly from model to model but the essential elements of analyzing the problem, gathering the data, analyzing the data, generating solutions, evaluating consequences of solutions, and choosing a solution are crucial steps in any classical, cognitive model of decision making. Figure 6–1 gives a schematic example of a *probability–event chain.* In Figure 6–1, alternative solutions A, B, and C are listed. Each solution is then followed with a set of possible consequences resulting from that solution to the problem. The tree is taken further in that the probable outcome of each consequence of each alternative

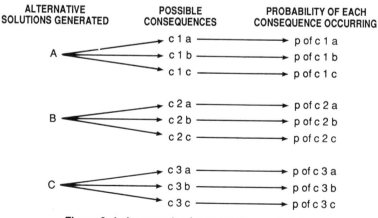

ALTERNATIVE SOLUTIONS GENERATED	POSSIBLE CONSEQUENCES	PROBABILITY OF EACH CONSEQUENCE OCCURRING
A	c 1 a	p of c 1 a
	c 1 b	p of c 1 b
	c 1 c	p of c 1 c
B	c 2 a	p of c 2 a
	c 2 b	p of c 2 b
	c 2 c	p of c 2 c
C	c 3 a	p of c 3 a
	c 3 b	p of c 3 b
	c 3 c	p of c 3 c

Figure 6–1. An example of a probability-event chain.

is then considered. Although the possible consequences and the probability of these consequences are separated in the diagram, they frequently occur simultaneously in the decision-making process. In other words, the manager would state, "If I choose alternative A, then the following will probably happen." Predicting consequences and the probability of these consequences occurring requires that the manager have a good deal of solid information about the problem and the alternative solutions that are being generated. For some types of decisions, for example, those involving fiscal issues where costs can be accurately predicted, the generating of possible and probable consequences may be more concrete. For other issues, for example, anticipating the reaction of individuals, consequences may be very difficult to predict. Figure 6–1 illustrates three possible consequences generated for each alternative solution; this is purely for diagrammatic purposes. In reality consequences may be greater or less in number.

A NORMATIVE MODEL OF DECISION MAKING

In the work of Vroom and Yetton (1973), as well as in the work of Vroom and Jago (1974), we find a normative model for decision making by both individuals and groups. Vroom and Jago " . . . view decision-making as a social process with the elements of the process presented in terms of events between people rather than events that occur within a person" (1974, p.247). Table 6–1 presents the *decision-making process* for both individual and group problems as defined by Vroom and Jago. Figure 6–2 illustrates the *decision process flow chart* for both individual and group problems. To use the decision flow chart illustrated in Figure 6–2, the manager must first state the problem and then answer the questions at the top of the figure regarding the problem. For example, if the answer to question **A,** "Is there a quality requirement such that one solution is likely to be more rational than another?", is "NO," the flow chart line leads us to question **D,** where a small black node indicates that we must pose question **D** about the problem.

Question **D** asks, "Is acceptance of decision by subordinates critical to effective implementation?" If the answer to this questions is "NO," the decision flow chart leads us to number **one.** Number **one** at the bottom of the figure indicates a feasibility set for both G = Group problems and I = Individual problems. For a Group decision the ideal solution would be A1 and a similar solution is indicated for an Individual decision.

In Table 6–1 we see the A1 solution defined as follows: "You

TABLE 6–1. THE DECISION-MAKING PROCESS

For individual problems		For group problems	
AI	You solve the problem or make the decision yourself, using information available to you at that time.	AI	You solve the problem or make the decision yourself, using information available to you at that time.
AII	You obtain any necessary information from the subordinate, then decide on the solution to the problem yourself. You may or may not tell the subordinate what the problem is, in getting the information from him. The role played by your subordinate in making the decision is clearly one of providing specific information which you request, rather than generating or evaluating alternative solutions.	AII	You obtain any necessary information from subordinates, then decide on the solution to the problem yourself. You may or may not tell subordinates what the problem is, in getting the information from them. The role played by your subordinates in making the decision is clearly one of providing specific information which you request, rather than generating or evaluating solutions.
CI	You share the problem with the relevant subordinate, getting his ideas and suggestions. Then *you* make the decision. This decision may or may not reflect your subordinate's influence.	CI	You share the problem with the relevant subordinates individually, getting their ideas and suggestions without bringing them together as a group. Then *you* make the decision. This decision may or may not reflect your subordinates' influence.
GI	You share the problem with one of your subordinates and together you analyze the problem and arrive at a mutually satisfactory solution in an atmosphere of free and open exchange of information and ideas. You both contribute to the resolution of the problem with the relative contribution of each being dependent on knowledge rather than formal authority.	CII	You share the problem with your subordinates in a group meeting. In this meeting you obtain their ideas and suggestions. Then, *you* make the decision which may or may not reflect your subordinates' influence.
DI	You delegate the problem to one of your subordinates, providing him with any relevant information that you possess, but giving him responsibility for solving the problem by himself. Any solution which the person reaches will receive your support.	GII	You share the problem with your subordinates as a group. Together you generate and evaluate alternatives and attempt to reach agreement (consensus) on a solution. Your role is much like that of chairman, coordinating the discussion, keeping it focused on the problem, and making sure that the critical issues are discussed. You do not try to influence the group to adopt "your" solution and are willing to accept and implement any solution which has the support of the entire group.

From Vroom and Jago. Decision making as a social process, Decision Sciences, 1974. Decision Sciences is published by the American Institute for Decision Sciences.

solve a problem or make the decision yourself, using information available to you at that time." In other words, a problem that does not require a solution that is likely to be more rational than another, and that does not require acceptance by subordinates as critical to its implementation, can be solved by managers making the decision themselves. The reader can use the decision

A. Is there a quality requirement such that one solution is likely to be more rational than another?
B. Do I have sufficient information to make a high quality decision?
C. Is the problem structured?
D. Is acceptance of decision by subordinates critical to effective implementation?
E. If I were to make the decision by myself, is it reasonably certain that it would be accepted by my subordinates?
F. Do subordinates share the organizational goals to be attained in solving this problem?
G. Is conflict among subordinates likely in preferred solutions? (This question is irrelevant to individual problems.)
H. Do subordinates have sufficient information to make a high quality decision?

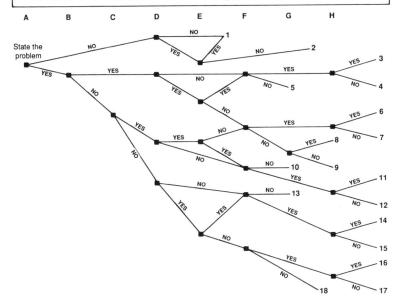

The feasible set is shown for each problem type for Group (G) and Individual (I) problems.

1. G: A1, A11, C1, C11, G11
   I: A1, D1, A11, C1, G1
2. G: C11
   I: D1, G1
3. G: A1, A11, C1, C11, G11
   I: A1, D1, A11, C1, G1
4. G: A1, A11, C1, C11, G11
   I: A1, A11, C1, G1
5. G: A1, A11, C1, C11
   I: A1, A11, C1
6. G: G11
   I: D1, G1

7. G: G11
   I: G1
8. G: C11
   I: C1, G1
9. G: C1, C11
   I: C1, G1
10. G: A11, C1, C11
    I: A11, C1
11. G: A11, C1, C11, G11
    I: D1, A11, C1, G1
12. G: A11, C1, C11, G11
    I: A11, C1, G1

13. G: C11
    I: C1
14. G: C11, G11
    I: D1, C1, G1
15. G: C11, G11
    I: C1, G1
16. G: G11
    I: D1, G1
17. G: G11
    I: G1
18. G: C11
    I: C1, G1

Figure 6–2. Decision process flow chart. *(From Vroom and Jago. Decision making as a social process, Decision Sciences, 1974. Decision Sciences is published by the American Institute for Decision Sciences.)*

process flow chart to follow more complex answers regarding the problem statement and come up with various feasibility sets for each problem as indicated in Figure 6–2.

The decision processes specified for each problem type are not arbitrary. The specification of the feasibility set of decision processes for each problem type is governed by a set of ten rules that serve to protect the quality and acceptance of the decision by eliminating alternatives that risk one or the other of these decision outcomes. (Vroom and Jago, 1974, p. 249)

For a more detailed discussion of the rules underlying the feasibility sets, the reader is referred to the work of Vroom and Yetton (1973) and Vroom and Jago (1974).

LIMITATIONS OF DECISION-MAKING MODELS

Rational, cognitive, and normative models of decision making have their place as helpful tools for the nurse manager. However, we must be aware of the reality of the limitations in the use of such decision-making models. The capacity of humans for processing information is relatively small and it may not be possible for a person to simultaneously consider all of the alternative solutions to a given problem.

> Given this limited capacity, even for familiar information, an individual has great difficulty trying to simultaneously consider all the available alternative solutions to a problem. Each choice has attendant outcomes and probabilities of success. To try to gather all the requisite information and then to juggle the trade-offs among all the variables at one is simply an impossible task for a human being. (Hatvany, 1982, p. 22)

Herbert Simon described this phenomenon in 1957 and termed it *bounded rationality*. Because the nurse manager is faced with solving complex problems in organizations and because all managers are limited as human beings by bounded rationality, they tend to search for ways of simplifying the problem into manageable sets of possible alternatives. In other words, nurse managers will develop their own model of reality to deal with the phenomenon of bounded rationality.

> The organizational and social environment in which the decision-maker finds himself determines what consequences he will anticipate, what ones he will not; what alternatives he will consider, what ones he will ignore. (March and Simon, 1958, p. 130)

Hatvany finds limitations and inadequacies in all of the phases of decision making. A discussion of these limitations may prove helpful by alerting the manager to the shortcomings of the process.

Problems in Information Gathering

The making of a rational decision with the use of a classical model of decision making is heavily dependent on accurate information. We have noted earlier the manager's preference for oral communication over written communication (Mintzberg, 1973). The manager obtains oral information from many sources both inside of and outside of the immediate organization. A nurse manager receives information from the staff, from superiors, and as a boundary-spanning person, and has input from outside of the organization that may affect decision making.

Hatvany cautions, however, that because oral information is subject to a great deal of distortion, the manager may not be receiving the best quality of information from these sources. Social psychology experiments (Downs, 1967) illustrate that information content is altered by a 98 percent loss if it is passed through a six-level hierarchy of people. This finding has made its way into a parlor game in which a message is whispered from one person to another and the initiator of the message and the final recipient of the message then compare the actual message, usually to the great amusement of those present when the degree of distortion is revealed. Although distortion of verbal information may be amusing for a parlor game, it has serious implications when one realizes that many managers depend heavily on oral communication for information gathering.

Another distortion in the gathering of information may come from the reluctance of subordinates to give managers bad news. This may be thought of as the "shoot the messenger" phenomenon. A subordinate may fear confronting the manager with negative information because he or she feels it may reveal his or her own failures or inadequacies. By eliminating vital facts, a subordinate may paint a brighter picture than is real for the manager.

A third problem in the information-gathering phase of decision making is something that has been termed *satisficing* (March and Simon, 1958).

Most human decision-making, whether individual or organizational, is concerned with the discovery and selection of *satisfactory alternatives;* only in exceptional cases is it concerned with the discovery and selection of *optimal alternatives.* To optimize requires processes several orders of magnitude more complex than those required to satisfice. An example is the difference between searching a haystack to find the sharpest needle in it and searching the haystack to find a needle sharp enough to sew with. (March and Simon, 1958, p. 141)

And so we see that managers in making decisions do search for alternatives, and examine alternatives carefully. As soon as a satisfactory alternative is found, however, the search usually ends and the manager stops searching with the first satisfactory alternative that is found. The manager thus has limited the search for alternatives and has *satisficed* rather than *optimized* in generating alternative solutions.

A similar phenomenon to satisficing is described by Braybrook and Lindbloom (1963) and is termed disjointed incrementalism or the science of muddling through. Disjointed incrementalism points out that decisions tend to be made in small, incremental ways rather than on a large scale. This phenomenon suggests that decision makers only examine solutions that are very similar to policies or situations that already exist and are in effect in the organization. How often, within the nursing organization, we can see examples of decisions in which satisficing or disjointed incrementalism was the phenomenon present. However, we as nurse managers are not alone in our inability to get beyond our own bounded rationality and look for optimizing solutions rather than ones that satisfice.

Problems in Evaluating Alternatives

In this phase of decision making, *suboptimizing* is one of the problems. Suboptimizing refers to the tendency to look at all of the alternatives at the same time, and in only one dimension, rather than examining each alternative one at a time and completely (Simon, 1977, pp. 39–81). For example, a health maintenance organization considering the setting up of a satellite clinic will have choices to make regarding the location of the new facility. Dimensions, such as the size of the site, its geographical location, and the expense involved in moving to such a location, are all elements that might be considered. If management considered all sites just on the basis of size and then perhaps selected the largest one without looking further at other dimensions of the decision, they would be suboptimizing. Suboptimizing tends to eliminate alternatives because of one dimension. It is dependent on the order in which the various dimensions are considered. Thus, a satellite clinic location might be selected merely because of size in the example given.

Bolstering is a social psychological phenomenon that has consequences for the decision-making process. Bolstering refers to the tendency that human beings have of dwelling on the positive consequences of a decision, which may in reality have both pos-

itive and negative consequences. Although the bolstering phenomenon can occur after a decision is made, it can also occur when
a decision is imminent. Thus, if we make a selection of one alternative solution, we tend to reinforce the positiveness of the
consequences of that decision. "This tendency to selectively avoid
information that contradicts a chosen course of action helps an
individual feel satisfied with a choice . . . " (Hatvany, 1982, p.
24).

Perseverance of ideas, even in the light of new information,
can be a problem in the decision-making process. The old cliché,
"First impressions are lasting," epitomizes the problem of per-
severence of ideas. When managers making a decision are presented with information, they often will try to explain that information. If, for example, a nurse manager is given a negative
report about one of the staff, he or she may actively seek to
explain the reasons for the negative report. Even in the light of
new information that contradicts the initial report, the manager
may continue to view that employee in a negative light.

Commitment to choices already made is another pervasive
phenomenon in decision making. It is often difficult for managers
to change their minds about decisions they have made, even in
the light of new evidence that suggests that these decision should
be reevaluated. This is especially true if the decisions were made
public. After a decision is made it sets a sequence of events into
motion. If the decision involved setting a tremendous amount of
organizational machinery into motion, or spending money, there
may be real constraints to changing one's mind. Thus, we begin
to make a psychological commitment to the decision we have
made, and may be reluctant to change our minds, even if perhaps
we should.

> This psychological commitment to the decision serves a valuable
> purpose during the unstable, early days of implementation. It
> serves no good purpose if it causes the manger to ignore warn-
> ing signals or become more committed to a choice by pouring
> in additional resources. . . . (Hatvany, 1982, p. 25)

Problems in Evaluating Probability Estimates

Because managers rely heavily on oral information and like the
vivid, easy, and enjoyable flow of information that comes ver-
bally, they may tend to ignore statistical information in making
probability estimates. Managers frequently use convenient heuristics, or ways of discovering things, such as *representativeness*,
availability, and *anchoring* (Hatvany, 1982, pp. 26–28). These
three phenomena, or heuristics, can be helpful in the decision-

making process but also may result in biases in the estimation of probability.

Representativeness is the phenomenon whereby a manager uses statistics that seem to make sense, rather than relying on hard, factual data. For example, if the ability to repay a loan is equally related to a person's income level and to the price of the shoes that he or she buys, one would tend to use income level as the predictor of repayment because it seems more representative of the ability to pay than does the price of the shoes, which may not seem realistic.

Another statistical concept that is hard to grasp and is easily replaced by more colorful explanations of events is *regression toward the mean*. "We may learn about tall fathers having shorter sons in statistics class, but we really expect the predictor of an outcome (height of fathers) and the outcome itself (height of sons) to be equally extreme. This simply makes 'better sense' " (Hatvany, 1982, p. 26).

Another problem in representativeness is the reliance on data from very small samples. A manager may look at a small sample of data and assume that the sample is representative of a much wider population. In doing research we may be very careful to have an adequate sample size, however, in the decision-making process, managers may find themselves heuristically relying on small samples to draw general conclusions.

Availability of explanations is another problem in predicting probabilities. Events or explanations that come to mind easily are deemed more likely to happen than those that do not come to mind, simply because these events are more available to our consciousness. The phenomenon of availability causes lessons that we have learned in the past to be deemed more likely to recur in the future than those events that have not occurred. It becomes easy to see, therefore, how the availability of images or explanations in our consciousness affects our ability to estimate what the probable outcomes of decisions will be (Hatvany, 1982).

The *vividness of information* tends to have a more substantial impact on decision making for the manager than does accurate statistics. Consider, for example, the news coverage that gives vivid detail of crimes committed in a large city. The vividness of these images may do more to influence a person's decision to travel to that city than would the actual statistics, which may rate the city at a moderate level in terms of crime.

Or suppose, for example, that you have decided to purchase a new car and have researched mileage, price, and have reviewed consumer reports that rate a particular foreign car as mechanically superior. On the basis of your research you have decided to purchase a particular car. In the meantime, however, you attend a party where there is a discussion about various cars and their advantages. You announce that you are buying a particular foreign car. One of the guests at the party reacts in disbelief and proceeds to tell you in vivid detail the problems that he had with just such a car. Mechanical breakdowns and expensive repairs and a near accident led him to sell the car after a few years. Do you believe that this encounter would affect one's decision to buy that particular car? Social psychology experiments have shown that *certain events presented in a framework of vivid and easily imagined stories are deemed more likely to occur than the same events that are presented in statistical or isolated information formats.* The preference of managers for verbal reports in gathering information for decision making makes them prey to this phenomenon.

Anchoring is another heuristic that may be used in making probability estimates. When making an estimate we naturally use a starting point or anchor from which to base our estimate. Adjustments should be made as we reach a final estimation, but frequently the adjustment is insufficient. For example, if we ask what percentage of people in the United States are 55 or older, and give the choices as 50 percent or more or less, 25 percent or more or less, 75 percent or more or less, we will find that those given the higher percentages as anchor will end up with too high an estimate, whereas those given the lower percentage as anchors will end up with too low an estimate. If one were to judge the probability of success in the use of primary nursing in an organization, the estimates of probable success might be too low if institutions where primary nursing was unsuccessful were used as anchors. An estimate of the probability of success would be too high if only institutions where it had thrived were used as anchors. Another problem related to anchoring is the phenomenon of judging the probability of a number of events occurring together. We tend to overestimate the probability of things happening at the same time because we think of them happening together, and view the probability of each one occurring as equal.

> In sum, heuristics are more often extremely useful. For example, it is clearly reasonable to use the availability of an event in memory as a rough guide to its frequency of occurrence. However, availability is affected not only by frequency; when availability is affected by imaginability also, using this convenient heuristic can lead to mistaken conclusions. (Hatvany, 1982, p. 28)

Keeping in mind that these limitations and problems occur in all phases of the decision-making process, we will examine some ways to avoid these pitfalls.

AVOIDING SOME OF THE PITFALLS IN DECISION MAKING

Gathering Information

The nurse manager should strive to get as much accurate information as possible. It must be observed that all the data that a manager is privy to is not necessarily valuable information for decision making. A manager must learn to examine the available data and extract that information that is essential for the decision-making process. Nurse managers have it within their scope of responsibility to design reporting systems that will allow them to monitor their organization carefully. These reporting systems should have built-in signals about the level and quality of the care being given, and about the functioning of the organization. If nurse managers do not build signals into their reporting system, they may spend a great deal of time studying reports that indicate that all is well within the organization. "It is a better use of time to manage 'by exception' and react only to signals that all is not well" (Hatvany, 1982, p. 29).

Reporting systems lend themselves to data that is easily quantifiable. It is easy for the nurse manager to design reports that will indicate staffing and scheduling patterns, turn-over and budgeting aspects of the organization. One of the problems with quantifiable data, however, is that this data can be manipulated. The nurse manager requires other systems of obtaining information with built-in signaling levels that indicate when trouble is brewing. This so-called soft information can be obtained through verbal and observation techniques. The manager's preference for verbal communication has already been noted. The manager should not abandon this vehicle of communication but should strive to make it systematic and comprehensive. An open door policy and frequent touring of the units are also important ways for nurse managers to gather information. A visit to a nursing unit and the sight of harried nurses, short-tempered aides who are surly to patients, call-lights buzzing, and staff speaking in angry voices to each other is a much clearer sign of problems and low morale on a unit than a census or staffing report from that unit could indicate. Nurse managers need to use their own observations to gather information, as well as relying on standardized reporting systems.

Evaluating Alternatives

We have discussed the problems of satisficing, suboptimizing, and disjointed incrementalism in the process of evaluating alternatives. The manager must be aware of all of these problems in the human decision-making process. The critical role of the *order of alternatives* must also be kept in mind. The tendency to select the first satisfactory alternative must be guarded against. If nurse managers are aware of this tendency, they can avoid selecting the first alternative that seems satisfactory and examine in detail other alternative solutions to the problem. Nurse managers should keep in mind, however, that the *limitations in the decision-making process should not paralyze the decision-maker.*

> The piece-mealing, remedial incrementalist or satisficer may not look like an heroic figure. He is nevertheless a shrewd, resourceful problem-solver who is wrestling bravely with a universe that he is wise enough to know, is too big for him. (Lindblom, 1968, p. 27)

There are times when nurse managers will find that a full, exhaustive use of the rational decision-making model is not necessary. The managers should be able to assess the problem and apply the decision-making approach that is most appropriate. For example, they may wish to use as rational as possible a method for fundamental organizational decisions such as policy decisions, salary decisions, major financial decisions, and major human resource decisions. Other problems may be solved then in a more incremental way, using a model with which the manager feels comfortable.

Probability Estimates

Estimating probability is aided by the use of *decision trees*, which force the expression of probability estimates. In making major decisions the nurse manager may wish to use a decision tree model. If the decision maker is aware of the major heuristics discussed here, they are less likely to be used when they are not appropriate. For example, people use less heuristics, or rules of thumb, in making decisions when they are placed in roles, such as jurors, that demand a rational decision-making process. It is illegal, for instance, for a bank loan to be approved by the person who helps you fill out the appliation, thereby preventing biases and encouraging rational decisions.

Finally, in estimating probability, some formal statistical training will be helpful to the nurse manager. Understanding statistics and being able to use them appropriately will help the nurse manager to avoid the inappropriate use of representativeness more successfully.

Selection of a Decision-Making Model

To make intelligent decisions nurse managers must not only be aware of the limitations in the decision-making process, but should also have a conception of the decision-making model they use. Explaining the way in which a decision is made is sometimes difficult. "In such a case, another approach may be tried: Simulating the decision-maker's model by examining the information gathered by the decision-maker and the choice to which this information led" (Hatvany, 1982, p. 31).

This process may, for example, show that the decision maker is making routine decisions based on quantitative data, such as staffing and scheduling patterns, or admission of students based on grade point averages and GRE scores. If so, these decisions may then be made in a routine way that does not require the decision-maker's full attention to each individual case. In routine situations, guidelines for decisions can be drawn up and then processed by subordinates. Routine decisions can also be made with the assistance of computers. Freeing managers from the boring repetitiveness of making routine decisions allows them to reflect more fully on the long-term goals of the organization and allows more time for creative, novel approaches and solutions to some of the more interesting problems that face the organization.

> While completely rational decision-making may not be possible, or even always necessary, an explicit, testable model that can be communicated to peers and subordinates will always serve the manager well. (Hatvany, 1982, p. 31)

THE USE OF COMPUTERS IN DECISION MAKING

The burgeoning use of microcomputers in nursing has great impact on the future of decision making in the nursing organization. Nurse managers can now have at their fingertips valuable data, quickly processed by the microcomputer, that relates to both human and fiscal resources. Many excellent software packages for use by both microcomputers and mainframe computers are available to assist nurse managers in making decisions about staffing the organization and the always difficult problems of scheduling and budgeting.

Most managers will find that the money spent for a micro-computer and some applicable software is easily recouped in the time saved by nurse managers in making repetitive, routine decisions in their organizations. Computers are also excellent tools for filing and managing data and have the capability of retrieving data in various formats for assistance in the decision-making process. For example, personnel files, which indicate licensure status, certification status, and special professional training, can be stored on a disc. The nurse manager then has the immediate ability to generate reports about the various kinds and levels of certification of the staff, without time consuming searching of files for this information. It is important for the computer novice to understand that one need not become a computer programmer to effectively use microcomputers or mainframe computers in the nursing organization. An understanding of what the computer can do and the kinds of software available that may be beneficial to a manager and the organization is a place to start. An introductory course in the use of microcomputers and the use of the specific software purchased are all that is usually necessary for the astute nurse manager to make effective use of computers in routine decision making.

We cannot hope in this chapter to cover all of the information a nurse manager would need to know to use a microcomputer in the decision-making process. We can, however, urge nurse managers to explore the literature regarding computers in nursing to determine in what ways the use of computers would be of assistance in the routine and complex decisions of their organization. The body of literature about computers in nursing is growing daily, as is the availability of innovative software. Lack of familiarity with computer technology should not deter nurse managers from exploring this important avenue of decision-making assistance. Opportunities to learn to use computers and software abound in the general community, as well as in the nursing community. Astute nurse managers will make use of these opportunities to advance their management skills.

REFERENCES

Allison, G. *Essence of decision*. Boston: Little, Brown, 1971.

Braybrooke, D., & Lindbloom, C.E. *A strategy for decision*. New York: Free Press, 1963.

Dewey, J. *How we think*. New York: Heath, 1910.

Downs, A. *Inside bureaucracy*. Boston: Little, Brown, 1967.

Hatvany, N. Decision making: Managers and cognitive models. In D. Nadler, M. Tushman & N. Hatvany (Eds.). *Managing organizations*. Boston: Little, Brown, 1982.

Janis, I., Mann, L. *Decision making: A psychological analysis of conflict, choice and commitment*. New York: Free Press, 1977.

Lindblom, C. *The policy-making process*. Englewood Cliffs, N.J.: Prentice Hall, 1968.

March, J., & Simon, H. *Organizations*. New York: Wiley, 1958.

Mintzberg, H. *The nature of managerial work*. New York: Harper & Row, Pub., 1973.

Simon, H. *The new science of management decision*. Englewood Cliffs, N.J.: Prentice Hall, 1977.

Vroom, V., & Jago, A. Decision making as a social process: Normative and descriptive models of leader behavior. *Decision Sciences*, 1974, 5.

Vroom, V., & Yetton, P.W. *Leadership and decision-making*. Pittsburgh: University of Pittsburgh Press, 1973.

PART II

Managing Fiscal Resources

CHAPTER 7

Managing Nursing Resources Through Patient Classification Systems

Ruth R. Alward

The most significant recent development to assist the nursing manager in allocating human resources according to perceived patient care needs is the evolution of patient classification systems (PCSs). Although these systems can, and no doubt will, increasingly be applied to long-term care as well as to community and outpatient settings, most of their development has occurred in acute-care hospitals in the United States and Canada over the past 40 years.

Nurses have long realized the inadequacy of using only a standard number of nursing hours per patient day as a guide to unit staffing on a daily basis. Unless a unit has an unusually homogeneous patient population, such as one might find in a normal newborn nursery or perhaps in a postpartum unit, 30 patients in one day will often require a great deal more or less nursing care than a different set of 30 patients just a day later. Patient classification systems were developed to help the nurse manager quantify this different in nursing care requirements, thus partially replacing subjective staffing judgments with objective ones.

In addition to differences in patient needs for nursing care, it should be remembered that the total nursing resource requirement and the resulting staffing levels are influenced by:

- The philosophy of the nursing organization
- The goals and objectives of the nursing organization
- Standards of nursing care and nursing practice
- Quality of nursing care to be delivered
- Cost and budgetary restraints
- Nursing staff's education, experience, and preferences
- Supportive services available to the nursing staff
- Medical practices
- Interdisciplinary cooperation
- Structure of the nursing organization
- Physical facilities and layout
- Unit sizes
- Availability of equipment and nursing supplies

This is by no means an exhaustive list of the variables the nurse manager must consider when staffing a unit. If a PCS is to be accepted as a valid basis for staffing and budgeting, all of these factors and more must be considered when the system is designed and as it is adapted for each individual nursing unit.

Classification of patients is not new. The health care system has through the years used medical diagnoses and treatment, age, and sex to differentiate categories of patients. The diagnosis related groupings (DRGs) used for determining prospective payments to be made by the federal government and other third-party payers are illustrative of current patient classification schemes based on these criteria. Other common classifications are more descriptive of the acuity of illness or the location where care is provided (e.g., intensive care, long-term care, home care).

When the term *patient classification* is used by nurses now, however, it usually refers to the use of an instrument to categorize patients according to the acuity of illness, the severity of symptoms, their degree of nursing dependency, the nursing interventions required during a specific period of time, or most likely, to some combination of these criteria. The variable of interest is the amount of nursing care required by the typical patient in a particular category, class, or level, and not the acuteness of the medical condition per se. Therefore, the use of the term *patient acuity systems* should be avoided in the context of classifying patients according to their need for nursing care. A patient can be acutely ill and not require as much nursing attention as a chronically ill patient who is more dependent for help with activities of daily living, requires more teaching, or has greater psychosocial needs. Medical terms and diagnoses have no consistent relationship with the amount of nursing care required and can be misleading if used in referring to PCSs used by nurses to match resources with demands.

When reference is made to a patient classification *system*, the use of a classification instrument has been combined with quantification of specific nursing interventions or categories according to the average nursing time required. It is this quantification aspect of PCSs that makes them useful to nurse managers for so many aspects of staffing and budgeting, not the classification by itself. It is the quantification aspects of a PCS that are difficult to develop and validate, although the reliability of the classification scheme is also necessary to the validity of the system.

Because development of a valid and reliable PCS is so difficult, it is very probable that fewer acute-care hospitals would have been interested in such a system were it not for pressure from the Joint Commission on Accreditation of Hospitals, beginning in the 1970s. The interpretation of Nursing Services Standard III states: "The nursing department/service shall define, implement, and maintain a system for determining patient requirements for nursing care on the basis of demonstrated patient needs, appropriate nursing intervention, and priority for care" (JCAH, 1983, p. 64). Furthermore, JCAH guidelines specify that a patient classification system is a major component of a staffing system used to determine nursing needs. A few nurse executives have resisted implementation of a PCS, fearing the legal implications of staffing deficiencies exposed by the system, but there is no evidence that lawsuits have resulted from the use of this management tool or influenced the results of legal action taken against nurses.

USES FOR PATIENT CLASSIFICATION SYSTEMS

The primary purpose of a PCS is to establish an objective method of response to the frequent changes in the amount of nursing time required for the nursing care of a particular patient population. Patient needs, as *perceived* by the nurse using the classifying instrument, are matched with the available nursing resources and staffing changes are initiated if the unit is either overstaffed or understaffed. (No claims can be made that the classifying instruments are sensitive to patient's *actual* needs for nursing care.)

A workload index can be produced for a given time period (usually a day or a shift) on each unit by dividing the required nursing hours by the actual nursing hours available. The workload index can be either predictive or retrospective.

$$\text{Predictive workload index} = 100 \times \frac{\text{Nursing hours required (by PCS) for the next shift or next day}}{\text{Scheduled nursing hours for same period}}$$

$$\text{Retrospective workload index} = 100 \times \frac{\text{Nursing hours required (by PCS) for past shift or day}}{\text{Actual nursing hours worked during same period}}$$

Examples of predictive workload index
A. Understaffing Example

$$\text{Workload index} = 100 \times \frac{\text{200 nursing hours required (PCS)}}{\text{150 nursing hours scheduled}} = 133\%$$

B. Overstaffing Example

$$\text{Workload index} = 100 \times \frac{\text{105 nursing hours required (PCS)}}{\text{150 nursing hours scheduled}} = 70\%$$

If the PCS is valid and reliable, the basic information generated can be helpful to the nurse manager in a variety of ways. Used predictively, the PCS guides daily adjustments in the staffing levels and encourages the creative use of nursing resources by making nurse managers continuously aware of excess or deficient staffing. It fosters use of variable staffing techniques, such as float pools and on-call, part-time staff, and directs help to units with the greatest patient care requirements. Furthermore, basing staffing adjustments on PCS objective data can decrease the time nurse managers spend on the time-consuming staffing function. Staffing clerks are often taught to make daily adjustments based on PCS results. Another predictive use of a PCS is to help balance staff members' workloads when making patient care assignments, especially in settings where primary nursing is not the mode of the care delivery. In the ideal nursing world, admission scheduling could also be based on predicted nursing unit workload indices, but, in practice, this seems to be the exception rather than the rule.

Unfortunately, many hospitals use PCSs only retrospectively rather than both predictively and retrospectively as intended by system designers. Perhaps this is because their nurse managers have not developed ways to respond quickly to changing patient care needs. Nursing staff members expect to receive assistance when a predictive PCS shows that they are significantly understaffed. If this expectation is repeatedly unfulfilled, the incentive decreases for accurate and continuous classification. On the other hand, nurses should also expect to be involved with interunit temporary transfers, cancelled temporary staff, or other procedures the nursing organization has developed to deal with overstaffing when it is shown by the PCS.

Common uses for retrospective PCS information are: justification for the nursing budget, justification for changes in the table of organization, and justification for the use of overtime and temporary staff. Most importantly, the data generated by a PCS over a period of time clearly demonstrate trends in the amount of nursing care needed by patients on a particular nursing unit. An analysis of workload indices over this period of time helps the nurse manager decide whether nursing vacancies should be filled or left open temporarily. As length of stay shortens, census days decline, and financial resources get scarcer, objective PCS data to support staffing levels become more urgent. If cyclical scheduling patterns are used, PCS data provide a way to evaluate the effectiveness and efficiency of these patterns over time and clues to improving the patterns as well. Retrospective workload indices can also be correlated with nursing quality indices for the same time periods.

When the PCS is used retrospectively to document actual nursing care delivered, it can be used as the basis for variable nursing charges to the patient's bill, as practiced by St. Luke's Medical Center in Phoenix, for more than a decade and described by Higgerson and Van Slyck (1982). In the limited number of hospitals that use variable billing for nursing services, the nursing charges are usually based on the number of days the patient was classified at each level or the number of points of nursing care provided each day of hospitalization. It is important to keep in mind that charges for nursing care cannot be based on predicted needs for nursing care but only on care actually delivered. Therefore, predictive data used for staffing future shifts cannot be used for charging purposes.

The State of Maine now requires hospitals to show nursing charges on all patient bills as a separate item from room and board charges. This makes the nurses more accountable for the costs and outcomes of nursing care as well as establishing the nursing department as a revenue-producing service. It is anticipated that more states will adopt this charging system and that PCSs will be used to document actual nursing care delivered.

With the advent of prospective payment by third-party payers in today's health care system, there is increased interest in analyzing the cost of nursing care as it relates to each DRG. A valid and reliable PCS is the logical foundation for this analysis as has been demonstrated at Strong Memorial Hospital by Sovie and her colleagues (Sovie, Tarcinale, Vanputte, and Stunden, 1985).

TYPES OF PATIENT CLASSIFICATION INSTRUMENTS

Abdullah and Levine (1965) identified the two most common types of patient classification instruments as based on either prototype or factor evaluation. Although today there are many variations of these two types, most patient classification instruments can still be subsumed under these heading.

The *prototype* evaluation instrument provides key descriptors of the typical patient in each category (Table 7–1). Patients are assigned to the category that best describes their conditions and the nursing care required. To be eligible for a category, patients need not meet all of the characteristics or require all

TABLE 7–1. PROTOTYPE CLASSIFICATION INSTRUMENT:
Medical–Surgical Units

Category I	Category II
1. Minor clinical symptoms	1. In early stages of chronic illness/ convalescing
2. Little or no deviation from normal behavior pattern	2. Occasional deviations from normal behavior patterns
3. Little or no activity restrictions	3. Activities limited or periodically restricted
4. Simple treatments and few medications	4. Treatment, observation, or instructions at least once each shift
5. Minimal supervision of self-care	5. Patient and/or significant others require periodic reassurance and support in acceptance of illness, condition, or level of disability

Category III	Category IV
1. Acute symptoms or disabling symptoms of chronic condition	1. Extremely acute symptoms/acutely or critically ill
2. Significant deviation from normal behavior patterns	2. Pronounced deviation from normal behavior patterns
3. Completely dependent on nursing personnel for activities of daily living	3. Requires total physical care
4. Frequent or complex treatments, observation, or instruction	4. Constant treatment, observation, and instruction
	5. Requires extensive emotional support

items of care listed. In some prototype systems, the descriptors are ranked by levels and the highest descriptor checked determines the category to be assigned. In general, classifying patients with a prototype evaluation instrument is a *best fit* rather than an *exact fit* process. The number of categories varies from three to as many as ten, with four or five the norm for medical–surgical classification instruments.

One of the main criticisms of the prototype instrument is the amount of subjectivity and ambiguity involved in classifying patients by means of this type of categorical scale. Detractors claim that although it allows some room for professional judgment, it also permits manipulation and error. Defenders of the prototype instrument are able to demonstrate that a high degree of interrater reliability is attainable if the scale has been well constructed, thoroughly explained to users, and is monitored for reliability on a continuous basis. (See *Reliability* section of this chapter for more detail.)

A *factor* evaluation instrument is one in which the points allocated for independently rated elements of nursing care or patient dependency are added. A category may be assigned on the basis of a patient's total points or number of check marks. Alternatively, the total points for the nursing unit's patient population may be converted to nursing care hours needed. Hanson (1983) subdivided factor instruments into those that provide a correlate index and those yielding a cumulative index.

The correlate index is obtained from factor evaluation instruments that list only a few carefully selected nursing activities and patients' characteristics, called critical indicators of care, that have been identified statistically as being highly correlated with a particular category (or amount) of nursing care. Although these instruments are short, and therefore, quickly completed, acceptance can be a problem unless the methodology is carefully explained and is understood by nurses using the system. There is a tendency for a brief instrument to be rejected because many aspects of nursing care and patient needs seem to be missing. It is hard for the staff nurse to comprehend that a single check mark in areas of bathing, ambulation, diet, intravenous therapy, dressings, and observations can establish a patient's category of care. "Where is the credit for my teaching and psychosocial care?" asks the nurse. A thorough explanation of the design of the correlate index answers this question. An example of a correlate index factor evaluation instrument is found in Table 7–2.

In contrast, the cumulative index is derived from a longer factor evaluation instrument that lists most of the frequently performed nursing care activities or patient characteristics and

TABLE 7–2. FACTOR CLASSIFICATION INSTRUMENT:
Correlate Index Type

Patient Classification	I	II	III	IV
Activity independent	( )			
Bath, partial assist		( )	( )	
Position, partial assist		( )	( )	
Position, complete assist			( )	( )
Diet, partial assist		( )	( )	
Diet, feed			( )	( )
IV add. q6h or more tko		( )	( )	( )
Observe, q1–2 h			( )	( )
Observe, almost constant				( )
Total	( )	( )	0.5	
Comments:				

From Alward. Journal of Nursing Administration, 13(2):14–19, 1983. Reprinted with permission.

needs. Points related to the average nursing time for completion of each item are totaled and translated into categories or nursing time required (Table 7–3). Although it takes longer to classify a patient using a cumulative index instrument, the nurses may feel that more of their effort is acknowledged with this system.

Another variation of the factor evaluation instrument uses relative value units (RVUs) to translate nursing activities into nursing time. As is true of so many aspects of PCS, there is no universal definition of a RVU. In the PCS described by Lewis and Carini (1984), a nursing activity or task that required, on average, less than 6 minutes to complete was assigned one RVU, tasks that took 7 to 12 minutes to complete were equated with two RVUs, and so on. After each patient's RVUs are added, this method allows calculation of the minimum (1 min × RVU) required for that patient's nursing care per shift as well as the maximum (6 min × RVU) time per shift. In this PCS, the RVUs are also designated according to the most fundamental skill level able to complete each nursing activity so that a calculation can be made of the nursing time required by a registered nurse, licensed practical nurse, or nursing assistant for each patient's care. In the Higgerson and Van Slyck (1982) methodology, RVUs were used to show the relationship between the levels of care (categories) and the actual cost of providing that care. Thus, for example, the relationship of category 1 to category 4 might be 1 RVU:3 RVU for a medical–surgical unit, showing that nursing costs each day are three times as much to care for the category 4 patient as for the category 1 patient.

TABLE 7–3. FACTOR CLASSIFICATION INSTRUMENT:
Cumulative Index Type—Patient Characteristics/Nursing Procedures

	Points
Admission	2
Feeds self without help	1
Feeds self with help	2
Total feeding	6
Tube/gastrostomy feeding—partial	1
Tube/gastrostomy feeding—total	4
Up with assistance	2
Bedrest	4
Partial bath	1
Total bath	2
Skin care	4
Incontinent	8
Partial immobility	4
Immobility	12
Isolation	4
Hypothermia	12
Extensive burns	12
Prepare for diagnostic test	2
Tube care	4
Intake and output	1
Special collection	1
Tracheostomy	3
Suction q3–4h	3
Suction q2h or more frequently	6
Irrigations/ostomies	3
O_2	2
IPPB	4
V/S q3–4h	2
V/S q2h or more frequently	6
Medications	1
IV	2
IV with medication	4
Teaching	6
Emotional	6
Language barrier	6
Sensory defects	6
Confused/disoriented	8
Unconscious	12
Discharge	1

Categories:
1   0–12 points
2   13–24 points
3   25–60 points
4   61–+ points
5   one-to-one care
Time value of points:
1 Point = 10 minutes

The most valued criterion in selecting the type of classifying instrument to be used in a PCS is acceptance by the staff and the managerial nurses who will be using it. Involvement in the selection and adaptation processes facilitates acceptance and on-going compliance. Interrater reliability has been demonstrated with both prototype and factor evaluation instruments as long as they are monitored on a routine but random basis after a thorough orientation for all users.

QUANTIFICATION OF PATIENT CLASSIFICATION SYSTEMS

In the previous section of this chapter, the instruments used to establish a category or level of perceived patient needs have been discussed. However, the essence of a PCS is not only the classifying instrument but also the quantification of factors and categories into nursing hours. Obviously, the primary purpose of using a PCS is not merely to decide *how many* patients on unit X are in categories 1 through 5, but to determine *the amount of nursing time* that should be allocated to the care of this group of patients on the next shift or perhaps to a similar group of patients next year.

Although there are many classifying instruments extant, differing in design and use, there is even greater variation in the way the factors or categories are quantified by assigning hours of nursing care per category or nursing minutes per factor. (This unfortunate lack of agreement on PCSs leaves nurse managers with only nursing hours per patient day, or perhaps in the future, with nursing hours per DRG, as a comparative nursing utilization statistic across hospitals.) No doubt the least satisfactory way to assign nursing hours to each category is to adopt the standards of another institution or standards published in the nursing literature. Whereas the classifying instruments can often be implemented with few changes by other units and other nursing departments caring for similar patients, calculation of valid standard nursing hours per category is a much more complicated process.

Because quantification of a PCS requires work analysis, knowledge, and skills more common to industrial and management engineers than to nurses, many nursing administrators purchase this expertise from a hospital association or management or nursing consulting firm. On-site nursing personnel, as well as the hospital's own management engineers, may also be involved in implementing the PCS, with or without assistance from outside consultants.

Work analysis techniques are the foundation of the patient classification quantification process. The nursing hours required to meet the projected needs of the average patient in each category (prototype or factor correlate instrument) or the average minutes required for each indicator of care or procedure (factor cumulative instrument) must be determined. For these analyses nursing personnel's time at work is divided into three components: (1) *direct time* spent with patients and their significant others, (2) *indirect time* spent on activities concerned with individual or collective patient care that is performed out of the patient's presence, such as taking report, preparing medications, care planning and conferences, charting and other documentation tasks, and (3) *nonproductive time* for personal activities and breaks, fatigue, and delays.

One way to collect the data from which to calculate the average direct and indirect nursing time spent on each category's typical patient is to observe a representative sample of nurses either on a continuous or intermittent schedule as they provide direct and indirect nursing care to patients in each category. Another data collection method involves having the nursing personnel themselves record all of their activities and how all of their working time is spent. This method allows large amounts of data to be quickly collected, saving time and money for the project, but it has been shown to be less accurate than the observational method (Williams, 1977). These methods can only be used if a classifying instrument has already been selected and implemented because they are concerned with identifying average nursing time required for each category of patient. The advantage of these methods is that the factors that give each nursing unit a unique organizational climate become part of the nursing standard hours per category. This can also be a disadvantage if quality of nursing care is low or if productivity on the unit is higher or lower than it should be, because these quantification methods are measuring how nursing time *was* spent during data collection periods and not how it *should* have been spent (Giovanetti and Thiessen, 1983).

The quantification method used by some consulting firms to implement a PCS is based on a comprehensive list of standard times for nursing tasks, to which is added an indirect nursing care constant for each patient day. If a unit under analysis is found to differ materially from the standard time in the time required by its personnel to perform a particular task, that task's standard time is adjusted. The indirect care constant should be developed to conform with unit practices. Convincing the nursing staff that this method is as valid as observational studies is often difficult. The advantage of this method is a shorter work analysis period and faster implementation of the PCS. Another alternative, usually too expensive, is classic time and motion studies concerned with all aspects of nursing care on each unit. With any of the work analysis methods, it is important to keep in mind that the standards calculated are averages and that individual patient's nursing care requirements will show variations from the mean.

In nursing organizations lacking the skills or financial resources to conduct work analysis studies for quantification of patient classification standards, it is possible to estimate nursing hours per category based on budgeted nursing care hours for a nursing unit, the projected number of patient days in each category, and the nurse manager's estimates of the proportional relationship of the workload represented by each of the categories. By using the percentage of nursing personnel assigned to each shift, the nursing standard per shift for each category is obtained (Table 7–4). Although the weakness of this method is an artificial relationship of the standard hours to the actual and perceived nursing care required by the average patient in each category, its strength is based on the reality of budgeted nursing hours in this health care climate of limited resources. If the data collection period was average in respect to patient care characteristics, the PCS will effectively detect shifts, days, weeks, months, or years with above or below average nursing care requirements so that corrections can be made in staffing levels (Alward, 1983).

The confidence that hospital administrators, nursing managers, and staff have in patient classification data is usually directly related to the way the quantification of category standards was approached. Agreement should be sought when the methodology is selected, and as the nursing standard hours per category are developed. Compatibility between the nursing budget and the staffing levels calculated using the PCS ensures the viability of the nursing organization's PCS.

VALIDITY AND RELIABILITY

Establishing and maintaining the validity and reliability of a PCS is difficult but essential. Staff and managerial nurses, hospital administrators, financial officers, and cost-based payers of health care bills must believe that the PCS actually and consistently measures what it claims to measure if staffing and budgetary

TABLE 7–4. USING THE NURSING BUDGET TO CALCULATE THE NUMBER OF NURSING HOURS FOR EACH PATIENT CATEGORY

Budgeted number of medical–surgical patient days next fiscal year = 10,400
Budgeted number of medical–surgical nursing hours per patient day (NHPPD) = 5.2
Budgeted number of medical–surgical nursing hours 10,400 × 5.2 = 54,080

Projected percentage of medical–surgical patient days in each category (from 3-month pilot period and other departmental considerations):

Category I = 10% of 10,400 = 1,040
Category II = 25% of 10,040 = 2,600
Category III = 50% of 10,040 = 5,200
Category IV = 15% of 10,040 = 1,560
100% 10,400 patient days

Percentage of nursing personnel by shift:
Days = 45%
Evenings = 35%
Nights = 20%

Budgeted number of nursing hours per patient day by category:

Category I (10%) 2 NHPPD × 1,040 = 2,080
Category II (25%) 4.5 NHPPD × 2,600 = 11,700
Category II (50%) 5.5 NHPPD × 5,200 = 28,600
Category IV (15%) 7.5 NHPPD × 1,560 = 11,700
Nursing hr = 54,080

Budgeted nursing hours per shift by category:

	Days	Evenings	Nights	Total NHPPD
Category I	0.45 × 2 = 0.9 nursing hr	0.35 × 2 = 0.7 nursing hr	0.20 × 2 = 0.4 nursing hr	2
Category II	0.45 × 4.5 = 2 nursing hr	0.35 × 4.5 = 1.6 nursing hr	0.20 × 4.5 = 0.9 nursing hr	4.5
Category III	0.45 × 5.5 = 2.5 nursing hr	0.35 × 5.5 = 1.9 nursing hr	0.20 × 5.5 = 1.1 nursing hr	5.5
Category IV	0.45 × 7.5 = 3.4 nursing hr	0.35 × 7.5 = 2.6 nursing hr	0.20 × 7.5 = 1.5 nursing hr	7.5

From Alward. Journal of Nursing Administration, 13(2):14–19, 1983. Reprinted with permission.

decisions, admissions, and patient charges are to be based on a PCS.

Validity

The validity of a PCS applies only to its use in a particular nursing setting, and, therefore, must be established on an individual unit basis. The generic question that must be answered for each unit is, "Does this PCS match perceived nursing care needs with available nursing resources?" The more specific questions are:

1. Is each patient placed in the category that best describes his or her needs for nursing care?
2. Do the nursing hours per category represent the average time needed to care for the typical patient in each category?
3. Can the budget support the level of nursing care required by the PCS?

If there are changes in nursing philosophy, standards of practice, nursing care delivery system, skill mix, treatments protocols, attending or house staff, physical facilities, equipment, supporting services, or other organizational characteristics, validity of the PCS can deteriorate. It must be assessed on a regular basis and quantification coefficients changed accordingly. Input from the unit nursing managers and staff is vital to the ongoing validity assessment. When it is obvious that changes have occurred in the nursing care delivery or the time required to care for patients, work analysis studies may again be necessary to establish new standard times for each category or indicator of care.

Reliability

Obtaining consistent results when different nurses classify a group of patients is the most important aspect of reliability related to PCSs. Clearly written guidelines should be available to each nurse user describing the procedure for classifying patients: the method, by whom, how often, and to whom reported. If a prototype instrument is used, examples of typical patients in each category should be given. Sample calculations should be provided for the entire process even though there may be computer or clerical support for some of the steps in the process.

Practice is using the classification instrument and calculating workload indices should be part of the nursing orientation program. In-service education on a periodic basis for all users helps to maintain an acceptable level of interrater reliability. It is not difficult to maintain the recommended 90 percent interrater reliability level if a regular weekly, or at least monthly, auditing process is followed, in addition to rigorous educational support. Clinical supervisors, clinical specialists, or other expert clinicians are often selected to reclassify a random selection of patients for comparison of their classifications with those of unit nurses. Frequent analysis of interrater reliability, studying how and where the rating differences occur, helps to identify inadequacies in the instrument and also to control *"category creep"* (padding patient care needs).

PROBLEMS IN IMPLEMENTING AND MAINTAINING A PATIENT CLASSIFICATION SYSTEM

Before implementing a PCS, there should be solid evidence that the nursing executive, middle management, and nurse user groups are committed to the system. Involvement throughout all stages of system development by many of those responsible for classifying patients and by nurse managers who will be using the staffing information provided, helps assure this commitment. Failures are numerous when a PCS is imposed on a nursing organization. This is especially true for systems with quantification standards that are not realistic for the institution. If the nursing hours per category are incompatible with the budget or with nurses' professional judgments, the system is more likely to fail.

The methodology used to quantify the categories must also be thoroughly understood by nurse users. For example, they should know how much indirect and nonproductive time was factored into the standards. Systems have been rejected by nurses because they did not know that an allowance for teaching and psychosocial nursing care had been added to each standard as the classifying instrument did not list these elements of care.

In a study that ranked 16 problems in planning and implementing PCSs, Huckabay and Skonieczney (1981) found that recruitment of nurses to meet staffing levels required by PCSs outranked by far the other problems. This study was conducted during a period of nursing shortage and similar stress can be expected to result today if the nurse manager is unable to staff at required nursing levels because of professional nurse shortage or increasing financial constraints. Staff complaints about the time and paperwork involved in classifying patients ranked second. The other stressors found in this study, ranked in declining order as problems to implementation of a PCS are:

- Feeling of stress in nursing staff
- Resistance to change

- Lack of reliability in classifying patients
- Resistance to classifying patients three times a day
- Difficulty in selecting a PCS
- Difficulty in conducting a research study (to select or test an existing PCS, work analysis studies)
- Feeling of stress in administrative nursing personnel
- Budgetary problems
- Cheating (padding patient care needs)
- Difficulty in motivating staff to implement PCS
- Lack of control by administration nurses
- Difficulty in training the in-service educators to do the PCS teaching
- Difficulty in motivating nursing administrators
- Difficulty in motivating hospital administrators

Knowing problem areas in advance helps the astute nurse manager deal with these concerns throughout the PCS planning, implementation, and maintenance phases.

The computer is another source of help for the nurse manager who relies on a PCS for management information. As more nursing management software has become available, an increasing number of nurse administrators are purchasing programs that facilitate patient classification system usage as well as assisting with staffing, scheduling, budgeting, and personnel control.

Although PCS data can be used to manually calculate unit staffing requirements, computer assistance becomes imperative if this data is later used to determine average nursing costs for each DRG. In many of the published methodologies (Shaffer, 1985), patient classification data are collected on each patient for each hospital day, along with the data used in grouping the patient into a specific DRG. By multiplying direct and indirect nursing costs for the average hour of nursing care, by the nursing hours delivered each day according to retrospective PCS data, the average nursing costs to care for each patient and each DRG in aggregate can be determined.

In summary, a PCS can be a great asset to top, middle, and first-line nursing managers. How valuable the information produced is depends largely on the validity and the reliability of the system, that is, the extent to which the PCS consistently and accurately measures: (1) perceived nursing care requirements for a group of patients for a given period of time and (2) the number of nursing hours required to provide this care.

Ideally, the PCS should be used both predictively as the basis for daily staffing of nursing units according to fluctuating patient care needs and retrospectively to support management

Example of Using PCS Data to Calculate Nursing Costs
For One Patient Stay

J. Smith	*DRG #357*	*Category*	*Standard Nursing Hours per Category*
	12/1/86	II	4
	12/2/86	IV	7
	12/3/86	III	5
	12/4/86	III	5
	12/5/86	II	4
			25 Nursing hours

Direct nursing costs per hour = $20.00
Indirect nursing costs per hour = 10.00
$30.00

25 hours × $30 =
$750 Nursing cost

decisions related to the use of nursing resources. Because of the many differences in patients, nurses, nursing organization units, and environments, assigning average time requirements for nursing care is at best an imprecise science. Moreover, PCSs are based on work analysis studies and skills unfamiliar to most nurses. They should be considered only as valuable adjuncts to rational staffing programs, informing the decisions of nurse managers without substituting for their professional and managerial judgments.

REFERENCES AND BIBLIOGRAPHY

Abdullah, F., & Levine, E. *Better patient care through nursing research.* New York: Macmillan, 1965.

Alward, R.R. Patient classification systems: The ideal vs. reality. *Journal of Nursing Administration*, 1983, *13* (2):14–19.

Giovanetti, P., & Thiessen, M. *Patient classification for nurse staffing: Criteria for selection and implementation.* Edmonton: Alberta Association of Registered Nurses, 1983.

Hanson, R.L. Predicting nurse staffing needs to meet patient needs. *Washington State Journal of Nursing*, 1976, *48*(3):7–11.

Hanson, R.L. *Management systems for nursing service staffing.* Rockville, Md.: Aspen Systems Corp, 1983.

Higgerson, N.J., & Van Slyck, A. Variable billing for services: New fiscal directions for nursing. *Journal of Nursing Administration*, 1982, *12*(6):20–27.

Huckabay, L.M.D., & Skonieczney, R. Patient classification systems: The problems faced. *Nursing & Health Care*, 1981, *2*,89–102.

Joint Commission on Accreditation of Hospitals. *A guide to JCAH nursing service standards.* Chicago: Joint Commission on Accreditation of Hospitals, 1983.

Lewis, E.N., & Carini, P.V. *Nurse staffing and patient classification.* Rockville, Md.: Aspen Systems Corp., 1984.

Shaffer, F.A. (Ed.). *Costing out nursing: Pricing our product.* New York: National League for Nursing, 1985.

Sovie, M.D., Tarcinale, M.A., Vanputte, A.W., & Stunden, A.E. Amalgam of nursing acuity, DRGs and costs. *Nursing Management,* 1985, *16*(3):22–42.

Williams, M.A. Quantification of direct nursing care activities. *Journal of Nursing Administration,* 1977, *7*(8):15–18.

CHAPTER 8

The Nursing Organization Budget: Basic Principles and Concepts

Robert Smith

In the current hospital environment it is imperative that nurse managers effectively manage not only clinical and human resources but the fiscal resources of the nursing organization as well. Complex financial environments impose strict demands for careful planning, requiring the accumulation and analysis of data measured to ensure the most cost effective use of personnel, supplies, and equipment while meeting patient care priorities.

The budget process focuses the dynamics of the environment, the overall organization, and the nursing organization into one fiscal policy. It involves assumptions based on historical data, in view of current goals and objectives to plan for the future. A budget can be viewed as simply a plan of what the job to be done is and what it will take to get the job done—with dollars attached. Nurse managers must be as articulate about the financial plan (i.e., budget) as they are about the clinical plan or they risk losing the running of their own "shop."

Historically, most nurse managers lacked formal education, training, or experience in financial matters. That picture has been changing as the financial pressures in health care have required everyone, nurses included, to become more cost conscious. Nurse managers must understand and learn how to use financial information in relating to other administrators and financial managers. Their credibility in budgeting and fiscal management will be as important an indicator of their stewardship as the quality of care their nurses provide. In fact, it may be one of the determinants of the quality of care their nurses provide.

One makes a serious mistake if the budget process is thought of as a once a year exercise in filling out forms for the accounting department. The budget should be a statement of policy. In reading through it one should be able to determine the priorities and direction of the fiscal period budgeted, usually 1 year. The budget should be a plan of what it will take to meet objectives in keeping with the policy directions. Plans, of course, are subject to change. The plan needs to be monitored throughout the fiscal period, both for changes made by decision, as well as changes not planned for. Expenditures need to be monitored and analyzed to determine if appropriate corrective action is necessary (over spending) as well as for the gathering of historical data to be used in future planning assumptions. Expenditure reports allow comparison between the plan (or budget) for the period, and the actual expenses for the same period. This analysis provides data useful in making better projections about future spending.

The budget process, then, is cyclical. From the time when the budget is being prepared, past performance is being analyzed to make better projections for the future. During the fiscal period, expenditure reports are being analyzed to compare against the plan, and as documentation of historical experience for future use. As planning time comes again, the cycle starts over.

If the budget process affords the nurse administrator the opportunity to identify and provide the resources necessary for quality patient care, it also accomplishes more than that.

Budgeting is certainly within the role of a nurse manager. It includes the basic steps in the classical approach to management crucial to fiscal resource management.

- **Planning.** This requires identification of options and choosing between them. Choices become decisions. Decisions become policy.
- **Communication and Coordination.** The budget process is a systematic way of communicating and coordinating efforts. It includes senior management, peer managers, junior managers, staff, and workers. It allows for input at each level. It necessitates the setting of priorities. It assists managers in coordinating uses of resources in view of budgeted goals and fosters efficiency.
- **Motivating.** By securing input from various staff members involved, there is opportunity to encourage them to take

a more active interest in the work environment. Participation in the planning stage facilitates implementation of the plan.

- **Controlling.** The monitoring and the analysis of expense reports on an ongoing basis permits taking responsible corrective action where indicated and when necessary. Decisions about over spending or underspending can be made while the problems are small, and before major problems result.
- **Evaluation.** The budget process allows measurement by comparison of assumptions or projections to actual performance.

It is imperative for the nurse manager to effectively manage the financial as well as the clinical and human resources of the nursing department. It is the budget process that permits the nurse manager to be an effective fiscal manager.

A *budget is a plan;* however, there are different types of planning processes hospitals and other organizations use.

The *strategic plan* is the organization's long-range plan for future survival. Senior management conducts analyses of various types to determine what the organization needs to best position itself to adapt to the changing environment. For a typical general hospital these would include:

- **Environmental Analysis.** Considers the geographics and demographics of the service area and patient population in view of changing factors and developing trends.
- **Service Analysis.** Considers number of beds per clinical service and their use now and in the future. Considers number of admissions, average length of stay, number of patient days, and so on.
- **Staff Analysis.** Considers medical staff by specialty; who are the major admitting physicians, their ages and tenure. Considers level and numbers of nursing staff needed for patient case mix and acuity.
- **Employee Relations Analysis.** Considers the hospital's ability to recruit and maintain staff needed at various levels: professionals, clericals, service employees. Considers what salary and benefit programs will allow them to remain competitive to attract the kinds of employees the hospital will need; what union labor contracts exist and when they expire.

- **Physical Plant Analysis.** Considers the age, condition, and improvements over the next 3 to 5 years. Considers what facilities need to be expanded or built (or demolished).
- **Quality Analysis.** Considers the hospital's strengths and weaknesses. Has the hospital shown a good track record in terms of accreditation and other inspection surveys?
- **Financial Analysis.** Considers various sources of income and how these might change in the next 3 to 5 years: investments, third-party reimbursers, and so on.
- **Legislative Analysis.** What is the impact of recently enacted laws relating to health codes and medical practice? What bills are now pending legislative action?
- **Political, Social Considerations.** What is the impact of these changes on the hospital's operations?

The strategic plan is very different from the day-to-day planning necessary to meet operational needs. It is concerned with long-range projections.

The *operational plan* is the shorter range plan (usually one fiscal year) for meeting day-to-day needs. Middle managers in nursing must identify specific goals to meet the objectives of the strategic plan for the coming fiscal year. They must determine what resources are necessary to implement the strategic plan for the coming fiscal period. The ability of the organization to develop an operational plan and to meet its operational goals helps to form the basis for future projections used in the development of the strategic plan. Senior management uses past performance in making decisions regarding future potential. The ability to meet current goals helps to determine future goals. One may think of operational performance as a major consideration in the development of a corporate strategy, which in turn, helps determine operational goals.

There are different planning needs for which to budget and there are different budget processes to meet those needs. There are different ways to construct a budget based on different needs and organizational preferences.

BUDGET PROCESSES

Historical or Incremental Budget

This method uses previous expenses, plus factors of change, to arrive at a new budget. The factors of change may include inflation, salary raises, and new program costs. The new budget is determined as an incremental cost over last year's budget. If last year's salary costs were $325,000 and a 5 percent raise is planned for the start of the fiscal year, then the increment over last year is $16,250 and the new salary budget is $341,250.

The historical method assumes that the history will be repeated (plus the 5 percent raise). It does not encourage a hard evaluation of what went into last year's $325,000 salary costs. Of course, the more history (data) you have available, the better able one is to project whether history will be repeated. Was last year's experience typical? Was it projected in the same fashion and how accurate was the projection compared to the original plan for last year?

Appropriations Budget

This method determines spending amounts (appropriated) that cannot be exceeded without an additional review process. It is generally a line by line authorization for specific items and specific amounts. It is also known as a *fixed* budget. It is most commonly used in governmental agencies.

Zero-Based Budget

This method requires total identification and justification of all expenses each year. It assumes nothing about previously approved programs and encourages a close examination of all levels of service.

The zero-based method has been found to be very time consuming from both the preparation and the review perspectives. Many programs can be assumed to be continuing if they have been approved as 2- or 3-year programs or as commitments to a permanent change. This method is most useful, however, in program budgeting when new program options are being prepared.

Program Budget

This method allows for identifying a smaller budget within a budget. In identifying a new program, this method allows for examination of all the costs *before* they are grouped together in the larger budget. Costs for salaries, equipment, and supplies for this program alone are separated out of the total budget for salaries, equipment, and supplies.

The program budget is useful in comparing and considering options for programs. It is especially useful when program costs transcend any one departmental budget, i.e, Nursing and Pharmacy setting up a Unit Dose system of pharmaceuticals supply on a nursing unit.

After the program is approved, the costs are then allocated to the appropriate budget categories in the respective departments.

Rolling Budget

This process allows for continuous updating of the budget plan within periods of the fiscal year. The fiscal year starts with one view of the budget but several months later may be modified in view of actual spending performance and revisions of cost projections. This may happen quarterly and forces a close analysis of each period as revisions for the next are due. This process encourages more accuracy because budgeting is being done closest to the period in which it occurs. Information tends to be harder. The rolling budget process requires much time by preparers and reviewers, but allows senior management the opportunity to shift priorities and identify trouble spots in spending within the fiscal year.

Trended Budget

This process is much like the historical budget process in that it relies on previous expense history to project the budget. Spending patterns from month to month are determined as they relate to the entire expenses for the fiscal year. These monthly spending percentages are then applied to the new budgeted amount. The spending patterns of previous years are trended forward, and dollars are apportioned in high and low spending months.

Comprehensive Budget

This process is not found in any textbook. Rather, it is a process that is actually an amalgam of all the others. Within any one total budget, there are expense categories that lend themselves to different types of budget processes. As we look at the budget building process in later chapters, you will discern the different techniques being used.

TYPES OF BUDGETS

Just as there are different planning needs and different budget processes, there are also different types of budgets. In a hospital nursing service, the nurse manager needs to be articulate and knowledgeable regarding two primary types of budgets: the capital budget and the operational budget.

Capital Budget

A capital budget is a plan for major outlays of money by an organization. It can be projected in concert with the operational budget and fiscal year, and in addition, be planned as a 3-year or a 5-year capital budget in conjunction with the strategic plan.

Items budgeted in a capital budget must cost at least as much as the organization's *definition of capital expense*. For example, some hospitals use a cutoff of $300.00. Capital items usually have a life expectancy of over 1 year. Capital expenses represent investments in the organization. Evaluating investments for capital purchase would include, but not be limited to, analyzing the answers to such questions as:

- Is the item needed as a replacement to maintain current levels of service?
- Is the item needed to provide an increased level of service?
- Is the item needed to provide a new service that does not exist currently?

The answers to these questions address the impact on revenue, patient care, personnel maintenance, as well as the cost and the life expectancy of the capital expense.

Each department prepares its wish list of capital requests, and these are reviewed by the hospital's executive board. A final, prioritized, capital budget list is approved based on the availability of capital funds.

Operational Budget

The operational budget is the day-to-day financial plan for a specific fiscal period, usually 1 year. It may be broken down into two distinct components: salaries for personnel and nonsalaries expenses for noncapital equipment and supplies. The budget process (preparation, monitoring, analysis) for salaries budgeting is covered in detail in the next chapter. The budget process for nonsalaries is covered in Chapter 10.

To prepare an operational budget, certain information is necessary. It is appropriate for an organization to issue a set of budget guidelines at the outset of the budget process. They are usually written by the vice president of finance with input from the vice president of human relations and materials management, as well as other members of the budget committee. Meaningful budget guidelines should include the following:

1. Statement of corporate strategy or long-range planning policy over the next several years.

2. Statistical data regarding patient census, patient mix, emergency room visits, clinic visits, patient days, average length of stay, and so on.
3. Salary programs with effective dates and amount to be budgeted for each category of personnel.
4. Nonsalary inflation guidelines secured by Purchasing Department from various suppliers for paper goods, metals, rubber, food, pharmaceuticals, and so on.
5. New programs, program changes, program deletions, e.g., expansion of operating rooms by second half of fiscal year and increase of operating room cases.
6. Budget calendar identifying holidays and budget periods (monthly/quarterly).
7. Forms: examples of forms to be used and how to complete them.
8. Review process with deadlines. A typical budget process could take 6 months.

Jan. 1	Guidelines issued
	Budget preparation by managers
Feb. 15	Initial submission to department heads
	Review by department head
	Presentation by managers to department head
	Revisions (approvals/deletions)
Mar. 15	Submission to administrator
	Review by administrator
	Presentation to administrator by department head
	Revisions (approvals/deletions)
Apr. 15	Submission to finance—budget director
	Review by budget director, vice president group
	Presentation to budget director, vice president group
	Revisions (approvals/deletions)
June 1	Submission to governing board
	Review by governing board
	Presentation to governing board
	Revisions (approvals/deletions)
June 30	Final budget approved
July 1	New fiscal year begins

No discussion of the budget process would be complete without an understanding of the financial structure of the organization. The financial structure consists of units that generate costs within the organization, commonly referred to as **cost centers.** Cost centers may be arranged for each department or there may be several within a single department. Nursing departments typically include a different cost center for each nursing clinical area, such as pediatrics, surgery, operating room, recovery room, or preferably for each nursing unit. Budgets are prepared for each cost center in a department and *rolled-up* as the nursing budget. Financial reporting follows the same cost-center arrangement so that the output (expense reports) can be readily compared to the input (cost-center budget). Cost-center budget and expense reports on a regular basis (i.e., monthly) provide important feedback regarding budget predictions and assumptions, as well as indications as to what actions may be necessary for responsible budget control. The cost-center arrangement also provides fiscal accountability in the organization.

TABLE 8–1. FINANCIAL STRUCTURE

Department Codes			
01	Administration	06	Laboratory services
02	Building services	07	Finance
03	Food services	08	Personnel
04	Radiology services	09	Purchasing
05	Nursing services	10	Security

Nursing Cost Centers		
Department	*Cost Center*	*Service*
05	01	Administration
05	02	Medicine
05	03	Surgery
05	04	Orthopedics
05	05	Operating room
05	06	Recovery room
05	07	Intensive care
05	08	Pediatrics

Personnel Codes or Salary Codes		Nonpersonnel Codes or Nonsalary Codes	
01	Management	10	Minor Medical Equipment
02	Professional	15	Medical Supplies
03	Aides	20	Pharmaceuticals
04	Clerks	25	Reprocessing
		30	Repairs

The salary of the head nurses in the ICU would be budgeted as 05-07-01.

The staff RNs in ICU as 05-07-02.

ICU medical supplies as 05-07-15.

As expenditures occur, each transaction would include the appropriate code to which the expense should be charged.

Monthly financial reports would list, for each cost center, the budget, the expenses, and the difference between the two (variance).

The financial structure, in addition to cost-center arrangements for accountability, includes a system of expense categories for groups of like items of expense. On the salary side, all management may be identified as one code, whereas clericals and service personnel would each be identified by their particular code. Budget input within a cost center would identify amounts needed for management and service personnel, as well as for clerical personnel assuming that there were all three types within a cost center. A professional code usually identifies nurses in a nursing department, pharmacists in a pharmacy department, social workers in a social service department, dietitians in a food service department, and so forth. On the nonsalary side, expense codes will differentiate between patient care supplies, office supplies, pharmaceuticals, minor equipment purchases, repair costs, travel and conference reimbursement expenses, and so forth. The ensuing chapters go into more detail regarding salary and nonsalary expense codes and the budget building process for each.

As dollars are expended, each organization must have a system for capturing expense transactions. Purchase orders to outside vendors, as well as interdepartmental transfers need to be recorded and reported so as to appropriately identify users or spenders. Tracking expenses for each item budgeted not only identifies spending patterns for historical reference, but also allows for identifying spending problems where responsible corrective actions may be necessary (Table 8–1).

REFERENCES AND BIBLIOGRAPHY

Althaus, J.N. Decentralized budgeting: Holding the purse strings: Part I and Part II. *Journal of Nursing Administration*, 1982, *12*(5): 15–20, *12*(6):34–38.

Beck, D. The departmental budgeting process. *The Health Care Supervisor* 1982, *1*(1):51–62.

Berne, R. Teaching budgeting: A basic course in public sector financial management. *Public Budgeting and Finance* 1982, *2*:111–122.

Boyer, C.M. Monitoring the budget—The personnel budget. *Journal of Nursing Administration*, 1983, *13*(6):35.

Carter, W.H., & Munack, L. Zero-based budgeting and program evaluation. *Journal of Rehabilitation*, 1977, 194.

Covaleski, M.A., & Dirsmith, M.W. Building tents for nursing services through budgeting negotiation skills. *Nursing Administration Quarterly*, 1984, *8*(2):1–11.

Dillion, R.D. Zero-based budgeting: An introduction. *Hospital Financial Management*, 1972, *27*(11):10–14.

Finkler, S. *Budgeting Concepts for Nurse Managers.* New York: Grune & Stratton, 1984.

Finkler, S.A. Electronic spreadsheets and budgeting: A case study. *Nursing Economics*, 1984, *2:*166–174.

Gleeson, S.V., Riddell, A.J., Yuneza, J.W., & Klane, E.M. The four P's of billing, credit, and collections for home health agencies. *Nursing Administration Quarterly*, 1984, *8*(2):74–81.

Moseley, O.B. Some thoughts on the human side of budgeting. *Supervisory Management* 1981.

Newton, R.L. Establishing a "rolling" budgeting process. *Hospital Financial Management*, 1981, *35*(5):54–56.

Ratkovitch, R. The nursing directors' role in money management. *Journal of Nursing Administration*, 1981, *11*(11):13–16.

Ruth, M.V., & Mohr, C.A. Budgeting in community health agencies. *Nursing Economics* 1984, *2:*47–50.

Schick, A.E., & Hatry, H. Zero-based budgeting: The manager's budget. *Public Budgeting and Finance.* 1981, *2:*82–87.

Schmied, E. Allocations of resources: Preparations of the nursing department budget. *Journal of Nursing Administration*, 1977, *7*(9):31–36.

Shapiro, S.E. ZBB–decision tool. *Hospital Financial Management*, 1977, *27*(10):40–43.

Sheedy, S., &Whitinger, R. Labor-based budgeting. *Nursing Management*, 1983, *14*(5):62–64.

Stevens, B.J. What is the executive's role in budgeting for her department? *Journal of Nursing Administration*, 1981, *11*(7):22–24.

Trofeno, J. Managing the budget crunch. *Nursing Management*, 1984, *15*(10):42–47.

Vanderzce, H., & Glusko, C. DRGs, valuable pricing and budgeting for nursing services. *Journal of Nursing Administration*, 1984, *14*(5):22–24.

Zegeer, L.J. Calculating a nurse staffing budget for a 20-bed unit at 100% occupancy. *Journal of Nursing Administration*, 1977, *7*(2):11–14.

CHAPTER 9

The Operational Budget of the Nursing Organization: Salaries

Robert Smith

A wide range of factors must be analyzed before a salaries budget can be built. This chapter discusses what each of these are, and demonstrates their use in budget building. For purposes of clarity, discussion and demonstration of the various factors relate to the preparation of an intensive care unit (ICU) salaries budget.

FACTORS IN BUILDING A SALARIES BUDGET

Analysis of the Guidelines for Relative Impact

Before beginning the budget preparation, it is important to read and analyze the budget guidelines. How do the policy statements and statistical data impact on the operations in the ICU? Will a planned increase in the operating room case load have an impact? What is the anticipated case load likely to be; does it make a difference if there are to be open-heart patients versus other types of patients? To the extent that the case load in the ICU will change, it may require a change in staffing of nurses, supplies consumed, or even equipment to be used. Development of staffing pattern in view of the patient mix, patient acuity, and hours of care required (at various skill levels) is the first step toward building a salaries budget. What skill levels and how many people at each level will it take to maintain the necessary staffing pattern?

Development of Staffing Pattern and Table of Organization

Nursing units require staffing 24 hours per day, 7 days per week, and 52 weeks per year. In the illustrations given in this chapter it is assumed that each full-time employee works 5 days per week, 8 hours per day with time off for earned vacation, holidays, and some sick leave. These benefits will vary from hospital to hospital, but for purposes of illustration, we will make certain assumptions as we develop the salaries budget. To the extent that these assumptions differ from your particular institution our numbers will be different; however, the concept remains the same. From the desired number of people that must be on duty each shift (and it could be different on days, evenings, and nights) and on any given day (and it could be different on weekends and weekdays, on holidays and regular days), it is possible to develop a table of organization, i.e., the number of *full-time equivalent* positions to be hired to provide the desired staffing pattern.

Program Change Justification

Once the table of organization is planned based on the need for the new fiscal year, it should be compared to the old table of organization. Changes should be identified and explained. Costs will later need to be attached to these explanations. If more personnel is needed as a result of an increase in the operating room case load, this should be identified as a program change. If they are needed because of changes in nursing practice, these additional costs should be tracked as a separate program. As the salaries budget is built, it is important to be able to track the additional cost (or savings) of any program changes being planned.

Actual Salaries of Current Staff

To build a salaries budget it is necessary to know the salaries of the current employees within each category of the cost center. This data is normally available on monthly expenditure reports detailing salary expenses. If there are position vacancies, there will be a need to budget salaries to the extent to which they may be filled. If historically ICU positions are all always filled, there will be a need to project when these current vacant positions will be filled. Transfers from other clinical areas of experienced nurses cost more in salaries than does the hiring of new nurses at beginning salary rates. Assumptions about these vacant positions need to be documented, so that as the fiscal year begins and expenditure reports are produced, they can be compared to the original assumptions and adjusted according to the actual performance.

Salary Scales and Increases

Once the actual salaries paid to current staff are known, and decisions are made about budgeting for vacancies, it is necessary to know what the salary scale will be for the various categories of employees. Will they change at some point in the new fiscal year? Will incumbents receive an increase different from the salary scale increase, or will the salary scales change at all? This information should be provided in the budget guidelines and may vary from year to year. Nurses on staff may receive an 8 percent increase, whereas the hiring scales may change by 5 percent. Service employees may receive a 5 percent increase, whereas the hiring scales do not change at all. The salary scales and increase programs need to be known to be planned for.

Shift Differential

Staff who work an evening shift or a night shift usually earn a shift differential bonus. Is this the same for the registered nurses as for the clerks or aides who work in the unit? Is the evening differential the same as the night differential? Is there a rotating shift differential paid to workers *not* on permanent shift that is different than that paid to those who are on permanent shift? How many shift positions are there? How many are filled by permanent shift employees versus rotating shift employees? Those data need to be known before any budget amount can be planned for shift differential.

Holiday Pay

Holiday differential is often paid to employees who work on the fixed holidays celebrated at a particular institution. Most institutions celebrate between 8 and 12 holidays. How does the staffing pattern change on holidays? Is it the same for Christmas and New Year's as it is for Washington's birthday? What is the additional pay due a worker on a holiday? Most institutions commonly pay one and a half times regular pay for working on a holiday. Because the first 8 hours are normally budgeted for every employee, those that work on the holiday will earn an extra 4 hours of pay. Where do the holidays fall in the monthly budgets?

How many people over three shifts will work on any given holiday at 4 hours of extra pay each, on 12 holidays per year?

Overtime

Overtime is a fact of life, especially in a nursing service where patient care priorities dictate the need to have staff to provide safe quality care. Overtime is usually paid at one and a half times regular pay. How many hours of overtime pay are required to be added to the budget? What are the criteria regarding overtime authorization? Is it incidental overtime (1 or 2 hours) or is it full-shift overtime to cover sick calls or vacancies? The nature and use of overtime hours should be analyzed before any budget for overtime is planned. It may be more efficient to add another position to the table of organization to reduce the full-shift overtime. This would be cost-effective. However, is the overtime mostly of the incidental type that would not be substantially reduced even if more positions were added? What has the overtime usage been over the past several years in view of the unit's turnover in the same period of time? Is there a relationship between the overtime pattern of expenses and the turnover experienced on the unit? What is the likelihood of this in the forthcoming fiscal period? Should we budget more overtime or less overtime?

Overtime can be one of the most closely examined items in the budget. It should be analyzed very carefully and efforts at reducing the need, and use, should be aggressive. Ignoring the expenses for overtime shows lack of planning and budget credibility.

On-Call Pay

On-call pay is commonly paid to nurses working in an operating room. What is the on-call pay policy of your institution? It could be half pay for on-call hours not at work, and one and a half time pay for on-call hours actually worked. What are the scheduled hours per week for on-call? Do all levels of staff take call or only senior staff (at higher pay rates)? How often have staff been called in to work? Will that be the same for the fiscal period for which the budget is being planned? What indicators are helpful in projecting on-call budgets?

Experience Differential

Experience differentials are salary programs designed to reward tenured and experienced staff. It is a common feature in teacher salary programs as well as in registered nurse salary programs.

What are the levels of experience rewarded, and what are the salary differentials paid at each level? How many nurses in your unit will be up for experience differential pay in the next fiscal year? At what points in the year will you need to budget how many increases? What was the total cost of your experience differential budgeted and actually paid last year? How close were your predictions? Current assumptions should be documented so as to be able to compare actual paid experience differential with amounts budgeted.

Promotional Increases

Promotional increases are paid to nurses as they move up the career ladder from staff nurse to senior staff nurse. How many levels of registered nurses does your institution have? What is the current number of nurses at the various levels? How much was paid in promotional increases last year? How much is the promotional increase at each step? How much do you need to budget for in the next fiscal year?

Turnover

What has the turnover been in the last fiscal year? How is it running in the current year to date? How soon have vacancies been filled in your unit? Has the average rate of pay of nurses in the unit gone up or down over the last several fiscal years (when adjusted for by salary raises)? Assumptions about turnover need to be documented and closely monitored as this is probably the single most unpredictable factor involved in budgeting salaries. How has the job market changed and what impact has that had or will have on your turnover? What steps have been taken to reduce turnover and how successful have they been? Can you quantify the turnover impact? Is the turnover seasonal? Can you adjust your budget dollars taking this into account?

Per Diem Nurses

Some hospitals have a flat per diem rate for nurses called in as *substitutes* for regularly scheduled staff. Per diem nurses are usually higher priced per hour than the regular staff, but as they receive no benefits (time off with pay or health insurance) they can turn out to be more cost effective in the long run. Because fringe benefits may not be reflected on most operational budgets, this last fact sometimes gets lost and per diem budgets appear more costly than they actually are. What is your unit's use of per diems? Do you have a cadre of per diems large enough to fill your needs? What are the criteria for calling in or scheduling per diems to work? How many shifts of per diems were budgeted and spent last fiscal year? How many are budgeted in the current fiscal year and how are the actual expenses running year to date? What staffing factors may influence your future use of per diems in the fiscal year being planned?

Fringe Benefits

The hospital must pay insurance companies for the cost of providing health insurance, life insurance, or any other type of benefits if offers its employees. These costs, as well as the cost of their benefits, i.e., tuition reimbursement, are referred to as fringe benefit costs.

In most hospitals the costs for fringe benefits are usually determined by the Personnel or Finance departments. They are usually stated in terms of a percentage of the gross salaries. The fringe benefits percentage rate would be included in the budget guidelines if individual departments are to include them in their budgets. Most often departments are not asked to budget for them; therefore, it is not included in this discussion.

BUILDING A SALARIES BUDGET

Having briefly raised some questions in discussing how various salary factors need to be analyzed, let us now turn to making some assumptions about each one and demonstrate how they may be used in developing a salaries budget for an ICU.

Staffing Pattern and Table of Organization

Given the patient population it has been decided that 20 nurses are needed on duty every day shift, 15 nurses on duty every evening shift, and 15 nurses on duty every night shift.

As every nurse gets 4 weeks vacation, 12 holidays, 12 sick days, and 2 days off every week, they will *not* work a total of 148 days per year. These *nonproductive* days are slightly different for the aides and clerks as they only have 2 weeks vacation per year. They will *not* work a total of 138 days per year. If the nonproductive days per year are subtracted from the total number of days per year (365), the nurses will actually work 217 days, whereas the aides and clerks will work 227 days each year. If the nonproductive days are divided by the actual number of work days, the relationship is 0.7 for RNs and 0.6 for the aides and clerks. For every one nurse on duty, an additional 0.7 must be hired; for every one aide or clerk on duty an additional 0.6 must be hired. For simplification the product has been rounded to whole numbers (Table 9–1).

TABLE 9–1. ICU—STAFFING PATTERN AND TABLE OF ORGANIZATION

Management
Supervisor RN
Day head nurse
Day assistant head nurse
Unit manager
Evening assistant head nurse
Night assistant head nurse

RNs

Staffing Pattern		$\times$ 1.7 =	Table of Organization		
20	day shift	$\times$ 1.7 =	34		
15	evening shift	$\times$ 1.7 =	25.5 = 26	rounded	
15	night shift	$\times$ 1.7 =	25.5 = 26	rounded	
50	**Total**		86	FTEs	

Vacations 4 weeks/year	=	20	days
12 holidays	=	12	days
12 sick days	=	12	days
2 days/week of	=	104	days
Total nonproductive days*	=	148	days

Total days in year	365
Minus nonproductive days	− 148
Actual number of days worked	= 217

$$\frac{\text{Nonproductive days}}{\text{Number of days worked}} = \frac{148}{217} = 0.68 = 0.7$$

For each one nurse, you need to add an additional 0.7 FTE

Aides

Staffing Pattern		$\times$ 1.6 =	Table of Organization		
day shift	6	$\times$ 1.6 =	9.6 = 10	rounded	
evening shift	5	$\times$ 1.6 =	8 = 8	rounded	
night shift	5	$\times$ 1.6 =	8 = 8	rounded	
			26	FTEs	

Clerks

day shift	3	$\times$ 1.6 =	4.8 = 5	rounded	
evening shift	2	$\times$ 1.6 =	3.2 = 3	rounded	
night shift	2	$\times$ 1.6 =	3.2 = 3	rounded	
	7		11	FTEs	

Vacations 2 weeks/year	=	10	days
12 holidays	=	12	days
12 sick days	=	12	days
2 days/week off	=	104	days
Total nonproductive Days	=	138	days

(Continued)

TABLE 9–1. (*Continued*)

Total days in year	365
Minus nonproductive days	– 138
Total number of days worked	= 227

$$\frac{\text{Nonproductive days}}{\text{Number of days worked}} = \frac{138}{227} = 0.6$$

For each one aide or clerk, you need an additional 0.6 FTE

ICU Current Table of Organization

		Management	RNs	Aides	Clerks	Total
Day	8–4:30 PM	4	34	10	5	53
Evening	4–12:30 AM	1	26	8	3	38
Night	12–8:30 PM	1	26	8	3	38
Total		6	86	26	11	129

*Note: Other nonproductive time may be factored into formula, i.e., continuing education days, committee meetings.

Program Change

Let us assume that after careful analysis of the increased operating room case load projected in the budget guidelines, i.e., number and types of additional cases, patient acuity, and nursing care hours needed, it has been determined that the staffing pattern will require two more nurses on the day shift, three more nurses on the evening shift, and three more nurses on the night shift. (The clinical formulas are omitted as we are mainly concerned with the *budget* impact of the program change.) To add the eight nurses to the daily staffing pattern, 13 more nurses must be hired (Table 9–2). The cost of these 13 nurses and their shift differential for evening and nights, as well as all the other salary factors to be looked, at need to be programmatically summarized as the impact cost for increasing the operating room case load. These projections are for a full fiscal year. As the full program impact will not take place until sometime later in the fiscal year, we will phase in the new positions as we anticipate filling them.

Actual Salaries

A computer run of active staff and their actual salaries usually can be secured from the Payroll department as an aid in budgeting. Otherwise, monthly activity reports should list salary data as well. In Table 9–3 the base salaries of the management staff currently total $204,000/year. Because we want to budget

TABLE 9-2. ICU—PROGRAM CHANGE
Additional Positions Due to Increase in Operating Room Case Load

Increase to Staffing Pattern			Increase to Table of Organization		Old Table of Organization		New Table of Organization	
2 (Day shift	8–4:30 PM)	× 1.7 =	3.4	+	34	=	37.4	= 37*
3 (Evening shift	4–12:30 AM)	× 1.7 =	5.1	+	26	=	31.1	= 31*
3 (Night shift	12–8:30 AM)	× 1.7 =	5.1	+	26	=	31.1	= 31*
8			13.6		86			= 99

Proposed ICU Table of Organization for New Fiscal Year

	Management	RNs	Aides	Clerks	Total
Day	4	37	10	5	56
Evening	1	31	8	3	43
Night	1	31	8	3	43
	6	99	26	11	142
Change	0	+13	0	0	+13

*Rounded

TABLE 9-3. ICU—ACTUAL SALARIES
Management

Day head nurse	$ 35,000	Fiscal year 7/1/86–6/30/87
Day assistant head nurse	32,000	Supervisor +6% effective 1/1/87
Evening assistant head nurse	30,000	Other management =5% effective 10/1/86
Night assistant head nurse	30,000	
Unit manager	32,000	
Sub total	159,000	
+ Supervisor	45,000	
	$204,000	Total base salaries at start of fiscal year

Average hourly rate calculations as follows:
July/August/September
  $204,000 ÷ 52 wk ÷ 40 hours ÷ 6 people = 16.35/hour

October/November/December
  159,000 + 5% = 7,950 = 166,950
  + Supervisor   =   45,000
                     211,950
  $211,950 ÷ 52 wk ÷ 40 hours ÷ 6 people = 16.98/hour

January through June
  Other management   = 166,950
  45,000 + 6% = 2,700 =   47,700
                   $214,650

  $214,650 ÷ 52 wk ÷ 40 hours ÷ 6 people = 17.20/hour

(Continued)

TABLE 9–3. (Continued)

July	22 days	×	8 hr	×	6 persons	=	1,056 hr	×	16.35	=	$ 17,266
Aug.	21 days	×	8 hr	×	6 persons	=	1,008 hr	×	16.35	=	$ 16,481
Sept.	22 days	×	8 hr	×	6 persons	=	1,056 hr	×	16.35	=	$ 17,266
Oct.	22 days	×	8 hr	×	6 persons	=	1,056 hr	×	16.98	=	$ 17,931
Nov.	21 days	×	8 hr	×	6 persons	=	1,008 hr	×	16.98	=	$ 17,116
Dec.	22 days	×	8 hr	×	6 persons	=	1,056 hr	×	16.98	=	$ 17,931
Jan.	22 days	×	8 hr	×	6 persons	=	1,056 hr	×	17.20	=	$ 18,163
Feb.	21 days	×	8 hr	×	6 persons	=	1,008 hr	×	17.20	=	$ 17,338
Mar.	22 days	×	8 hr	×	6 persons	=	1,056 hr	×	17.20	=	$ 18,163
Apr.	22 days	×	8 hr	×	6 persons	=	1,056 hr	×	17.20	=	$ 18,163
May	21 days	×	8 hr	×	6 persons	=	1,008 hr	×	17.20	=	$ 17,338
June	22 days	×	8 hr	×	6 persons	=	1,056 hr	×	17.20	=	$ 18,163
	260						12,480 hr				$211,319
							÷ 2080 = 6 FTEs				

hours as well as dollars, it makes sense to use an average hourly rate. Divide the total base salaries by 52 weeks, by 5 days a week, by six persons who work 8 hours each per day. The average hourly rate at the start of the fiscal year is then $16.35.

We have assumed that of the *current* table of organization of 86 RNs the average hourly rate for 80 currently active RNs (with 6 vacancies) is $13.50/hour (or $28,080/year). For the sake of brevity each of the 80 RNs and their respective salaries have not been listed.

There are usually at least two vacancies at any one time; therefore the budget is built for 84 RNs only. We determine not to budget the two vacancies at the average rate, as it is anticipated that they will be filled with lower paid nurses. The new total base salaries now brings the average hourly rate for RNs to $13.46/hour (Table 9–4). (The two vacancies not budgeted here will be budgeted elsewhere later.)

Our average hourly rate for aides is assumed to be $9.00/hour or $18,720/year at the start of the fiscal year.

Our clerks earn $8.00/hour at the start of the fiscal year. All employees work a 40-hour week.

TABLE 9–4. BASE SALARIES FOR REGISTERED NURSES

Table of organization	= 86	
	− 6	current average vacancies
	80	(actual average hourly rate = $13.50)
Scale = $26,500 ÷ 52 wk ÷ 40 hr	+ 4	(vacancies at scale = $12.74)
	84	RNs at 13.46/hour
		(2 vacancies *not* budgeted here)

TABLE 9–4. (*Continued*)

July

    80   RNs $2,246,400 ÷ 52 wk ÷ 40 hr ÷ 80 = $13.50/hour
    +4 RNs   106,000 ÷ 52 wk ÷ 40 hr ÷ 4 = $12.74/hour
    84       $2,352,400 ÷ 52 wk ÷ 40 hr ÷ 84 = $13.46/hour

August

    84 RNs $2,352,400
    +8 RNs   212,000 ($26,500 × 8)
    92 RNs $2,564,400 ÷ 52 wk ÷ 40 hr ÷ 92 = $13.40/hour

September

    92 RNs $2,564,400 + 5% = (+128,220) = $2,692,620
    _5 RNs   26,500 + 5% = (+1,325) 27,825 × 0.5 =   139,125
                                                               $2,831,745

    97 RNs $2,831,745 ÷ 52 weeks ÷ 40 hr ÷ 97 = $14.04/hr

July	22 days × 8 hr × 84 RNs =	14,784 hr × 13.46 =	$ 198,993
Aug.	21 days × 8 hr × 92 RNs =	15,456 hr × 13.40 =	$ 207,110
Sept.	22 days × 8 hr × 97 RNs =	17,072 hr × 14.04 =	$ 239,691
Oct.	22 days × 8 hr × 97 RNs =	17,072 hr × 14.04 =	$ 239,691
Nov.	21 days × 8 hr × 97 RNs =	16,296 hr × 14.04 =	$ 228,279
Dec.	22 days × 8 hr × 97 RNs =	17,072 hr × 14.04 =	$ 239,691
Jan.	22 days × 8 hr × 97 RNs =	17,072 hr × 14.04 =	$ 239,691
Feb.	21 days × 8 hr × 97 RNs =	16,296 hr × 14.04 =	$ 228,796
Mar.	22 days × 8 hr × 97 RNs =	17,072 hr × 14.04 =	$ 239,691
Apr.	22 days × 8 hr × 97 RNs =	17,072 hr × 14.04 =	$ 239,691
May	21 days × 8 hr × 97 RNs =	16,296 hr × 14.04 =	$ 228,796
June	_22 days × 8 hr × 97 RNs =	_17,072 hr × 14.04 =	$_ 239,691
	260	198,632 hr	$2,770,328
		÷ 52 wk ÷ 40 hr =	95.5 FTEs

Salary Scales and Increase Programs

Budget guidelines have announced salary increase programs to be budgeted as follows:

Senior management (Supervisor)	6%	effective Jan. 1, 1987
Other management	5%	effective Oct. 1, 1986
Professional staff (RNs)	5%	effective Sept. 1, 1986
Aides and clerks	5%	effective Jan. 1, 1987

In Table 9–3, the different months of the year are budgeted at different average hourly rates as the increase programs took effect in October and January, respectively. The same concepts would apply to the staff nurses, aides, and clerks.

TABLE 9–5. BASE SALARIES FOR AIDES AND CLERKS

Aides

Average hourly rate $9.00
plus 5% = .45
effective 1/1/87 $9.45/hour

Clerks

Average hourly rate $8.00
plus 5% = .40
effective 1/1/87 $8.40/hour

Aides

July	22 days × 8 hr × 26 =	4,576 hr × $9.00 =	$ 41,184
Aug.	21 days × 8 hr × 26 =	4,368 hr × $9.00 =	$ 39,312
Sept.	22 days × 8 hr × 26 =	4,576 hr × $9.00 =	$ 41,184
Oct.	22 days × 8 hr × 26 =	4,576 hr × $9.00 =	$ 41,184
Nov.	21 days × 8 hr × 26 =	4,368 hr × $9.00 =	$ 39,312
Dec.	22 days × 8 hr × 26 =	4,576 hr × $9.00 =	$ 41,184
Jan.	22 days × 8 hr × 26 =	4,576 hr × $9.45 =	$ 43,243
Feb.	21 days × 8 hr × 26 =	4,368 hr × $9.45 =	$ 41,278
Mar.	22 days × 8 hr × 26 =	4,576 hr × $9.45 =	$ 43,243
Apr.	22 days × 8 hr × 26 =	4,576 hr × $9.45 =	$ 43,243
May	21 days × 8 hr × 26 =	4,368 hr × $9.45 =	$ 41,278
June	22 days × 8 hr × 26 =	4,784 hr × $9.45 =	$ 45,209
	260 days	54,080 hr	$498,888
		÷ 52 wk ÷ 40 = 26 FTEs	

Clerks

July	22 days × 8 hr × 11 =	1,936 hr × $8.00 =	$ 15,488
Aug.	21 days × 8 hr × 11 =	1,848 hr × $8.00 =	$ 14,784
Sept.	22 days × 8 hr × 11 =	1,936 hr × $8.00 =	$ 15,488
Oct.	22 days × 8 hr × 11 =	1,936 hr × $8.00 =	$ 15,488
Nov.	21 days × 8 hr × 11 =	1,848 hr × $8.00 =	$ 14,784
Dec.	22 days × 8 hr × 11 =	1,936 hr × $8.00 =	$ 15,488
Jan.	22 days × 8 hr × 11 =	1,936 hr × $8.40 =	$ 16,292
Feb.	21 days × 8 hr × 11 =	1,848 hr × $8.40 =	$ 15,523
Mar.	22 days × 8 hr × 11 =	1,936 hr × $8.40 =	$ 16,262
Apr.	22 days × 8 hr × 11 =	1,936 hr × $8.40 =	$ 16,262
May	21 days × 8 hr × 11 =	1,848 hr × $8.40 =	$ 15,523
June	22 days × 8 hr × 11 =	1,936 hr × $8.40 =	$ 17,002
	260 days	22,880 hr	$187,614
		÷ 52 wk ÷ 40 = 11 FTEs	

TABLE 9–6. TOTAL BASE SALARIES FOR ICU

Management	$ 211,319
Staff nurses	2,770,328
Aides	498,888
Clerks	187,614
Total base salaries	$3,668,149

In Table 9–4, we can see that the fiscal year starts with the original table of organization of 84 (86 − 2 vacancies) RNs. We anticipate filling 8 of the new 13 positions in the second month (August) of the fiscal year, and the remaining 5 positions in the third month (September). We have determined that these five new positions will be filled at the hire scale, which also changes on September 1.

The first month, July, starts out with 84 positions at $13.46/hour (as assumed previously). In the second month, August, we budget for 84 plus 8 new positions at the old scale rate bringing the new average rate for all 92 NRs to $13.40/hour.

In the third month, September, we add the remaining five new RNs positions (92 + 5 = 97), which is still two positions short of the new table of organization of 99. We have phased in the hiring of the 13 new RNs in recognizing their availability and the impact of the increased operating room case load. Also, in September we want to give all current staff a 5 percent raise as well as increase the hiring scale by 5 percent at which the five new RNs will be hired.

See Table 9–5 for the base salaries for aides and clerks. Total base salaries are illustrated in Table 9–6.

Shift Differential

It is assumed that shift differential for management and staff RNs is the same: $3000/year for permanent evenings; $4000/year for permanent nights; and $2500/year for rotating rate. Given the ICU table of organization, it is assumed that budgeting every planned shift position at the permanent differential pay will be sufficient. Close monitoring throughout the previous year has resulted in an insignificant variance from that plan. Shift differential for aides and clerks is 10 percent of base salary. Table 9–7 shows calculations for shift differential for RNs.

Calculations can, depending on the need and time constraints, be gross, i.e., annual estimates for ballpark figures, or they can be detailed, based on weekly or monthly calculations to be used for budget input documents.

TABLE 9-7. SHIFT DIFFERENTIAL

Management	Evenings assistant head nurse	$3,000 ÷ 12 months =	$ 250/month
	Nights assistant head nurse	$4,000 ÷ 12 months =	$ 333/month
		$7,000	$ 583/month
			× 12
	Actual amount to be budgeted =		$ 6,996

Staff nurses	Evenings	31 × $3,000 = $ 93,000 ÷ 12 =	$ 7,750/month
	Nights	31 × $4,000 = $124,000 ÷ 12 =	$ 10,333/month
		$217,000 ÷ 12 =	$ 18,083/month
			× 12
	Actual amount to be budgeted =		$216,996

Aides   Evenings and nights:

7/1–12/31
16 aides × $9.00/hr × 40 hr/wk × 26 wk × 10% = $14,976
$14,976 ÷ 6 mo = $2,496/mo

1/1–6/30
16 aides × $9.45/hr × 40 hr/wk × 26 wk × 10% = $15,726
$15,726 ÷ 6 mo = $2,621/mo
              Total shift differential for aides = $30,702

Clerks   Evenings and nights:

7/1–12/31
8 clerks × $8.00/hr × 40 hr/wk × 26 wk × 10% = $ 4,992
$4,992 ÷ 6 mo = $832/mo

1/1–6/30
6 clerks × $8.40/hr × 40 hr/wk × 26 wk × 10% = $ 5,244
$5,244 ÷ 6 mo = $874/mo
              Total shift differential for aides = $10,236

SHIFT DIFFERENTIAL BUDGET	GROSS	DETAILED
Management	$ 7,000	$ 6,996
Staff RNs	217,000	216,996
Aides	30,700	30,702
Clerks	10,234	10,236
	$264,934	$264,930

For management and staff nurses, the shift differential amount is fixed per nurse, but will vary depending on the number of nurses for which we will be budgeting. Note that the fiscal year started (current table of organization, Table 9–1) with 26 nurses on evenings and 26 nurses on nights. It was later phased in 13 new positions, 5 of which were added to evenings and 5 of which were added to nights. We anticipated that of the 13 new positions, none would be hired in July, 8 would be hired in August, and the remaining 5 would be hired in September (see Table 9–4).

The base salaries budget was based on these assumptions. In building the shift differential budget, we did *not* factor the shift table of organization for these months, but rather used the new table of organization as if it were in effect from the start of the fiscal year. To that extent, there is some "fat" in our budget. Because we cannot really be sure which of the 8 nurses hired in August and which of the 5 nurses hired in September will be hired for evenings or nights, we have provided the money in the budget to take care of any combination. Indeed, we are not even 100 percent certain that all 13 new positions will be filled by our stated target assumptions. The important point here is to document assumptions, so that future performance reports can be compared to the plan for explanation of variances. It could have been said the 8 nurses hired in August would include 3 for evenings and 2 for nights, and the 5 nurses hired for September would include the remaining 2 for evenings and 3 for nights. The costing out of shift differential would then be more exact. The shift differential was not factored to simplify the example.

In calculating shift differential for the aides and the clerks, we must adjust the differential amount as the differential is paid as 10 percent of base salary. Because both categories of employees receive pay increases in January, the differential amounts will change in mid-fiscal year. The number of aides (or clerks) times their average hourly rate, times their number of hours per week, times the number of weeks at that rate, times the 10 percent increase, yields the shift differential amount needed for that period. As the rate changes, the calculation yields a different amount. For simplification, equal monthly amounts in the first 6 months, and different monthly amounts equally in the second 6 months have been budgeted. Table 9–8 summarizes the monthly shift

TABLE 9–8. MONTHLY SHIFT DIFFERENTIAL BUDGET

Month	Management	RNS	Aides	Clerks	Total
July	$ 583	$ 18,083	$ 2,496	$ 832	$ 21,994
Aug.	583	18,083	2,496	832	21,994
Sept.	583	18,083	2,496	832	21,994
Oct.	583	18,083	2,496	832	21,994
Nov.	583	18,083	2,496	832	21,994
Dec.	583	18,083	2,496	832	21,994
Jan.	583	18,083	2,621	874	22,161
Feb.	583	18,083	2,621	874	22,161
Mar.	583	18,083	2,621	874	22,161
Apr.	583	18,083	2,621	874	22,161
May	583	18,083	2,621	874	22,161
June	583	18,083	2,621	874	22,161
Total	$6,996	$216,996	$30,702	$10,236	= $264,930

differential budget necessary for all staff for the entire fiscal year. Expenditure reports detailing shift differential paid can easily be compared to the plan. Significant variances *can* be documented, both for future budgeting use and as an understanding of a monthly variance analysis.

Holiday Differential

Holiday differential must be budgeted in the months in which the holidays occur as significant spending variances can result if they are not.

Let us decide that the management staff do not earn additional pay for working on a holiday. They are usually off but simply earn an alternative day off if they should work.

Staff nurses, on the other hand, will earn one and a half times their regular pay. As the first 8 hours is already budgeted in base salaries, we will need to add an additional one half day or 4 hours of pay for every employee who works on a holiday.

It is assumed that staffing drops to 60 percent on all holidays. (We could further factor the budget by assuming that it will drop to 50 percent on Christmas and 50 percent on New Year's with all nurses having either one of the two holidays off.) For simplification, a 60 percent rate for all holidays is assumed. There are 12 holidays, but one holiday, July 4, falls out before the scheduled pay raise (for nurses) on September 1. Aides and clerks have scheduled pay raises on January 1. Holidays should be budgeted according to the salary rates we projected at the time the holiday pay is earned.

Table 9–9 lists the holidays celebrated and Table 9–10 shows how the holiday differential pay has been calculated for the nurses, aides, and clerks. Note that the nurses' calculations for July and September differ in the table of organization used and the average

TABLE 9–9. HOLIDAY SCHEDULE

July	Independence Day
August	None
September	Labor Day
October	Columbus Day
November	Election Day, Veteran's Day, Thanksgiving Day
December	Christmas Day
January	New Year's Day, M. L. King's Birthday
February	Lincoln's Birthday, Washington's Birthday
March	None
April	None
May	Memorial Day
June	None

TABLE 9–10. HOLIDAY DIFFERENTIAL PAY

Management—None

Staff Nurses		Hours	Dollars
July—Table of Organization = 84 × 60% = 50.4 =	50 Nurses × 4 hr each 200 hr ×13.46/hr $2,692	 200	 $2,692
August—None			
September Table of Organization = 97 × 60% = 58.2 =	58 Nurses × 4 hr each 232 hr ×14.04/hr $3,257	 232	 $3,257
October—same as September		232	$3,257
November— 232 × 3 holidays =	696 hr		
$3,257 × 3 holidays =	$9,771	696	$9,771
December—same as September		232	$3,257
January— 232 × 2 holidays =	464 hr		
$3,257 × 2 holidays =	$6,514	464	$6,514
February—same as January		464	$6,514
March—none			
April—none			
May—same as September		232	$3,257
June—none			
	Total	2,752	$38,519

Aides		Hours	Dollars
July—Table of Organization = 26 × 60% = 15.6 =	16 Aides × 4 hr 64 hr × 9.00/hr $ 576	 64	 $ 576
August—none			
September—same as July		64	$ 576
October—same as July		64	$ 576
November—64 × 3 holidays =	192 hr		
$576 × 3 holidays =	$1,728	192	$1,728
December—same as July		64	$ 576
January—same as July New hourly rate	× 64 Aides × 9.45 $ 605		
64 × 2 holidays =	128 hr		
$605 × 2 holidays =	$1,210	128	$1,210

(Continued)

TABLE 9–10. (Continued)

Aides		Hours	Dollars
February—same as January		128	$1,210
March—none			
April—none			
May—6,44 × 1 = 64 hr			
$605 × 1 = $605		64	$ 605
June—none	Total	768	$7,057

Clerks

Table of Organization = 11 × 60% = 6.6 =

7 clerks per holiday
×   4 hr each   × 7 holidays =
28 hr   196 hr
×8.00/hr
$ 224 per   × 7 holidays =
holiday $1,568

Five holidays occur after the January 1 raise:

28 hr   × 5 holidays =
×8.40/hr   140 hr
$ 235

× 5 holidays =
$1,175
Total hr 196 + 140 = 336
Total dollars $1,568 + 1,175 =
$2,743

TABLE 9–11. HOLIDAY DIFFERENTIAL BUDGET

Month	Management	RNs	Aides	Clerks	Total
July	0	$ 2,692	576	224	$ 3,492
Aug.	0	0	0	0	0
Sept.	0	$ 3,257	576	224	$ 4,057
Oct.	0	$ 3,257	576	224	$ 4,057
Nov.	0	$ 9,771	1,728	672	$12,171
Dec.	0	$ 3,257	576	224	$ 4,057
Jan.	0	$ 6,514	1,210	470	$ 8,194
Feb.	0	$ 6,514	1,210	470	$ 8,194
Mar.	0	0	0	0	0
Apr.	0	0	0	0	0
May	0	3,257	605	235	4,097
June	0	0	0	0	0
	0	$38,519	$7,057	$2,743	= $48,319
Total hours		2,752	768	336	3,856

hourly rate applied. All remaining holidays are projected to cost the same; the monthly amounts vary depending on how many holidays occur in any particular month.

Note the calculations for the aides' holiday differential. Because the table of organization does not change in the fiscal year, the number of hours needed for each holiday is the same. The new average hourly rate is applied after the salary increase date of January 1.

In calculating the clerks' holiday differential budget, we took a shortcut; the table of organization never changes, so each holiday requires the same number of hours; the salary rate changes January 1. Because there are seven holidays before January 1, and five holidays after January 1, we can shorten the steps if monthly budgets are too time consuming. The monthly amounts can be determined from these calculations at a later time. Table 9–11 summarizes the holiday differential budget for the fiscal year.

Overtime

Overtime budgets can be a very sensitive issue. It is generally agreed that paying one a half times a salary to an employee working longer than a regular shift is expensive and not productive. To *plan* an overtime budget, in view of this, requires close analysis and solid justification.

There are valid reasons to authorize overtime on a nursing unit. Sick/absent calls may require overtime for staff to maintain a minimum staffing pattern for safe patient care. An increase in patient census or acuity may require staffing above the planned staffing pattern. The hours and reasons for overtime should be logged to analyze, over periods of time, whether additional positions would reduce the need for overtime. If the overtime is mostly in full shifts (8 hours), additional positions could cost less and be more productive (assuming these full shifts totaled one full-time equivalent (FTE)). If the overtime need is mostly incidental, i.e., a few hours never amounting to a full shift, then more FTEs may not be the answer. The overtime hours spent, the nature of the hours spent, the reasons for the hours spent, and the costs of the hours spent should be documented on an ongoing basis for periodic analysis.

Based on a review of our data, and what we know about the staffing plan for the new fiscal period, it is determined that the overtime will be budgeted as follows: management, none (they are exempt from overtime pay); staff nurses, four shifts per month; aides, two shifts per month; and clerks, one shift per month.

TABLE 9–12. OVERTIME BUDGET FOR STAFF NURSES

July	4 shifts × 8 hr =	32 hr	13.46 × 1.5 = 20.19	32 × 20.19 = $ 646
Aug.	4 shifts × 8 hr =	32 hr	13.40 × 1.5 = 20.10	32 × 20.10 = $ 643
Sept.	4 shifts × 8 hr =	32 hr	14.04 × 1.5 = 21.06	32 × 21.06 = $ 674
Oct.	4 shifts × 8 hr =	32 hr	14.04 × 1.5 = 21.06	32 × 21.06 = $ 674
Nov.	4 shifts × 8 hr =	32 hr	14.04 × 1.5 = 21.06	32 × 21.06 = $ 674
Dec.	4 shifts × 8 hr =	32 hr	14.04 × 1.5 = 21.06	32 × 21.06 = $ 674
Jan.	4 shifts × 8 hr =	32 hr	14.04 × 1.5 = 21.06	32 × 21.06 = $ 674
Feb.	4 shifts × 8 hr =	32 hr	14.04 × 1.5 = 21.06	32 × 21.06 = $ 674
Mar.	4 shifts × 8 hr =	32 hr	14.04 × 1.5 = 21.06	32 × 21.06 = $ 674
Apr.	4 shifts × 8 hr =	32 hr	14.04 × 1.5 = 21.06	32 × 21.06 = $ 674
May	4 shifts × 8 hr =	32 hr	14.04 × 1.5 = 21.06	32 × 21.06 = $ 674
June	4 shifts × 8 hr =	32 hr	14.04 × 1.5 = 21.06	32 × 21.06 = $ 674
Total budget		= 384 hr		= $8029

The staff nurses' overtime budget is illustrated in Table 9–12. For each month, the number of planned shifts is multiplied by the number of hours per shift, resulting in the total hours per month. These monthly planned hours should be compared to the amounts actually spent each month as the performance reports are generated.

Because overtime is paid at one and a half times the regular rate, we multiply the average hourly rate by one and a half to get the average hourly overtime rate. By multiplying the hours planned each month, by the average hourly rate for overtime pay, the amount of dollars to be budgeted each month is determined.

Note that the average rates of pay change in each of the first 3 months of the fiscal year. As a result, so does the amount of overtime dollars required. Our plan does not call for a difference

TABLE 9–13. OVERTIME BUDGETS FOR AIDES

July	2 shifts × 8 hr =	16 hr	9.00 × 1.5 = 13.50	16 × 13.50 = $ 216
Aug.	2 shifts × 8 hr =	16 hr	9.00 × 1.5 = 13.50	16 × 13.50 = $ 216
Sept.	2 shifts × 8 hr =	16 hr	9.00 × 1.5 = 13.50	16 × 13.50 = $ 216
Oct.	2 shifts × 8 hr =	16 hr	9.00 × 1.5 = 13.50	16 × 13.50 = $ 216
Nov.	2 shifts × 8 hr =	16 hr	9.00 × 1.5 = 13.50	16 × 13.50 = $ 216
Dec.	2 shifts × 8 hr =	16 hr	9.00 × 1.5 = 13.50	16 × 13.50 = $ 216
Jan.	2 shifts × 8 hr =	16 hr	9.45 × 1.5 = 14.18	16 × 14.18 = $ 227
Feb.	2 shifts × 8 hr =	16 hr	9.45 × 1.5 = 14.18	16 × 14.18 = $ 227
Mar.	2 shifts × 8 hr =	16 hr	9.45 × 1.5 = 14.18	16 × 14.18 = $ 227
Apr.	2 shifts × 8 hr =	16 hr	9.45 × 1.5 = 14.18	16 × 14.18 = $ 227
May	2 shifts × 8 hr =	16 hr	9.45 × 1.5 = 14.18	16 × 14.18 = $ 227
June	2 shifts × 8 hr =	16 hr	9.45 × 1.5 = 14.18	16 × 14.18 = $ 277
Total		192 hr		= $2,658

TABLE 9–14. OVERTIME BUDGET FOR CLERKS

July	1 shift × 8 hr = 8 hr	8.00 × 1.5 = 12.00	8 × 12.00 = $ 96
Aug.	1 shift × 8 hr = 8 hr	8.00 × 1.5 = 12.00	8 × 12.00 = $ 96
Sept.	1 shift × 8 hr = 8 hr	8.00 × 1.5 = 12.00	8 × 12.00 = $ 96
Oct.	1 shift × 8 hr = 8 hr	8.00 × 1.5 = 12.00	8 × 12.00 = $ 96
Nov.	1 shift × 8 hr = 8 hr	8.00 × 1.5 = 12.00	8 × 12.00 = $ 96
Dec.	1 shift × 8 hr = 8 hr	8.00 × 1.5 = 12.00	8 × 12.00 = $ 96
Jan.	1 shift × 8 hr = 8 hr	8.40 × 1.5 = 12.60	8 × 12.60 = $ 101
Feb.	1 shift × 8 hr = 8 hr	8.40 × 1.5 = 12.60	8 × 12.60 = $ 101
Mar.	1 shift × 8 hr = 8 hr	8.40 × 1.5 = 12.60	8 × 12.60 = $ 101
Apr.	1 shift × 8 hr = 8 hr	8.40 × 1.5 = 12.60	8 × 12.60 = $ 101
May	1 shift × 8 hr = 8 hr	8.40 × 1.5 = 12.60	8 × 12.60 = $ 101
June	1 shift × 8 hr = 8 hr	8.40 × 1.5 = 12.60	8 × 12.60 = $ 101
Total	96 hr		= $1182

in the monthly overtime needed, but if it did, the change would easily be factored in.

The concepts are the same for the aides and the clerks. Monthly overtime hours are planned based on authorized criteria for overtime, historical experience of overtime use, and plans for the future fiscal year. Tables 9–13 and 9–14 show how the overtime budget is built. Table 9–15 summarizes the overtime plan for this unit in *hours* and Table 9–16 in *dollars*.

It is important to note that once the plan is adopted, those who authorize overtime need to be aware of the plan and monitor the plan. Variances from the plan need to be explained each month as the performance reports are made available. Variance analysis helps support more accurate overtime needs for future budgeting as well as permit responsible corrective action as needs dictate.

TABLE 9–15. SUMMARY OF OVERTIME BUDGET—HOURS

Month	Staff Nurses	Aides	Clerks	Total
July	32	16	8	56
Aug.	32	16	8	56
Sept.	32	16	8	56
Oct.	32	16	8	56
Nov.	32	16	8	56
Dec.	32	16	8	56
Jan.	32	16	8	56
Feb.	32	16	8	56
Mar.	32	16	8	56
Apr.	32	16	8	56
May	32	16	8	56
June	32	16	8	56
Total	384	192	96	672

TABLE 9–16. SUMMARY OF OVERTIME BUDGET—DOLLARS

Month	Staff Nurses	Aides	Clerks	Total
July	$ 646	$ 216	$ 96	$ 958
Aug.	643	216	96	955
Sept.	674	216	96	986
Oct.	674	216	96	986
Nov.	674	216	96	986
Dec.	674	216	96	986
Jan.	674	227	101	1,002
Feb.	674	227	101	1,002
Mar.	674	227	101	1,002
Apr.	674	227	101	1,002
May	674	227	101	1,002
June	674	227	101	1,002
Total	$8,029	$2,658	$1,182	$11,869

On-Call Pay

On-call pay may be paid to nursing staff to assure their availability at times when they are not on duty. The operating room usually has an on-call arrangement for emergency operations at odd hours. The on-call pay policy provisions vary from organization to organization. Certain assumptions will be made to demonstrate the budget building steps. Table 9–17 states the on-call provisions and Table 9–18, the on-call calculations. The on-call policy does *not* apply to the ICU in our example.

Experience Differential

The records on experience differential due for the ICU nurses indicate that the supervisor as well as the head nurse and assis-

TABLE 9–17. ON-CALL BUDGET FOR STAFF NURSES

Assumptions

1. Schedule:	Mon.–Fri. 12 midnight–8 AM =	8 hr × 5 days	= 40 hour/week
	Sat. 12 midnight–8 AM		= 16 hour
		= 16 hours	
	Sun. same as Sat.		= <u>16</u> hour
			72 hour/week
2. Rates:	Home on-call = $^1/_2$ pay		
	In on-call = $1^1/_2$ pay—paid from time call		
	to time leaving hospital		
3. In on-call:	Average 10 hr/week		
4. Calendar:	Assume 5 wk (months Sept./Dec./Mar./June)		
	Assume 4 wk (months remaining)		

TABLE 9–18. ON-CALL BUDGET CALCULATION FOR STAFF NURSES

July	4 wk × 72 hr = 288 hr $\frac{1}{2}$ × \$13.46 = 6.73 288 × 6.73 = \$ 1938	
	4 wk × 10 hr = <u> 40 hr</u> 1$\frac{1}{2}$ × \$13.46 = \$20.19 40 × 20.19 = <u>\$ 808</u>	
	4 wk × 82 hr = 328 hr \$2746	
Aug.	4 wk × 72 hr = 288 hr $\frac{1}{2}$ × \$13.40 = \$ 6.70 288 × 6.70 = \$ 1930	
	4 wk × 10 hr = <u> 40 hr</u> 1$\frac{1}{2}$ × \$13.40 = \$20.10 40 × 20.10 = <u>\$ 804</u>	
	4 wk × 82 hr = 328 hr \$2734	
Sept.	5 wk × 72 hr = 360 hr $\frac{1}{2}$ × \$14.04 = \$ 7.02 360 × 7.02 = \$ 2527	
	5 wk × 10 hr = <u> 50 hr</u> 1$\frac{1}{2}$ × \$14.04 = \$21.06 50 × 21.06 = <u>\$ 1053</u>	
	5 wk × 82 hr = 410 hr \$3580	
Oct.	4 wk × 72 hr = 288 hr $\frac{1}{2}$ × \$14.04 = \$ 7.02 288 × 7.02 = \$ 2022	
	4 wk × 10 hr = <u> 40 hr</u> 1$\frac{1}{2}$ × \$14.04 = \$21.06 40 × 21.06 = <u>\$ 842</u>	
	4 wk × 82 hr = 328 hr \$2864	

Nov.	same as Oct. =	328 hr = \$ 2,864	
Dec.	same as Sept. =	410 hr = \$ 3,580	
Jan.	same as Oct. =	328 hr = \$ 2,864	
Feb.	same as Oct. =	328 hr = \$ 2,864	
Mar.	same as Sept. =	410 hr = \$ 3,580	
Apr.	same as Oct. =	328 hr = \$ 2,864	
May	same as Oct. =	328 hr = \$ 2,864	
June	same as Sept. =	<u>410</u> hr = <u>\$ 3,580</u>	
Total yearly budget	=	4,264 hr = \$36,984	

tant head nurse have completed the sequence of steps. They are not entitled to any further differentials. The evening assistant head nurse will be due a differential in September; the night assistant head nurse in March (Table 9–19).

The staff nurses will be due experience differentials as noted in Table 9–20. The summary for the experience differential budget is shown in Table 9–21.

Experience differential programs may vary. For purposes of illustration it is assumed that there are four experience levels:

TABLE 9–19. EXPERIENCE DIFFERENTIAL BUDGET FOR ASSISTANT HEAD NURSE

Evening, effective Sept. = 10 mo × \$25 each = \$250
Night, effective March   = 4 mo × \$25 each = <u> 100</u>
                     Total   \$350 as follows:

July	0	Jan.	\$25
Aug.	0	Feb.	\$25
Sept.	\$25	Mar.	\$50
Oct.	\$25	Apr.	\$50
Nov.	\$25	May	\$50
Dec.	\$25	June	\$50

TABLE 9–20. EXPERIENCE DIFFERENTIAL BUDGET FOR STAFF NURSES

July	6 × $25 = $150	Cumulative total amount per month = $ 150
Aug.	2 × 25 = 50	Cumulative total amount per month = 200
Sept.	4 × 25 = 100	Cumulative total amount per month = 300
Oct.	0	Cumulative total amount per month = 300
Nov.	1 × 25 = 25	Cumulative total amount per month = 325
Dec.	3 × 25 = 150	Cumulative total amount per month = 475
Jan.	0	Cumulative total amount per month = 475
Feb.	0	Cumulative total amount per month = 475
Mar.	2 × 25 = 50	Cumulative total amount per month = 525
Apr.	0	Cumulative total amount per month = 525
May	1 × 25 = 25	Cumulative total amount per month =

2 years, 4 years, 6 years, and 8 years. Each level pays an increase of $300 per year, or $25 per month.

Because of turnover, it may be assumed that several of the 20 staff nurses will resign in the course of the fiscal year (or perhaps even before its start), which would mean we would not need the entire $4950 budgeted for the staff nurse group. Vacancies, however, may be filled by transfers from four other units, and these nurses may or may not be due an experience differential while in the ICU. The experience differentials actually paid each month need to be logged so that any variance from the budgeted plan can be known and explained. It can be assumed from past experience that by budgeting for the known due differentials, our variance from the actual differentials paid in the past is so small as not to warrant any change in our budget assumption.

TABLE 9–21. EXPERIENCE DIFFERENTIAL BUDGET

Month	Management	Staff	Total
July	0	$ 150	$ 150
Aug.	0	200	200
Sept.	$ 25	300	325
Oct.	25	300	325
Nov.	25	325	350
Dec.	25	475	500
Jan.	25	475	500
Feb.	25	475	500
Mar.	50	525	575
Apr.	50	525	575
May	50	550	600
June	50	650	700
Total	$350	$4,950	$5,300

TABLE 9–22. PROMOTIONAL INCREASE TO STAFF NURSES

Month	To Staff Nurse II			To Staff Nurse III		Total	Monthly Total
July	2 × $50 = $100 =	100		1 × 100 =	100 = $	200	$ 300
Aug.	2 × 50 = 100 =	200		1 × 100 =	200 =	400	600
Sept.	2 × 50 = 100 =	300		1 × 100 =	300 =	600	900
Oct.	2 × 50 = 100 =	400		1 × 100 =	400 =	800	1,200
Nov.	2 × 50 =	500		1 × 100 =	500 =	1,000	1,500
Dec.	2 × 50 =	600		1 × 100 =	600 =	1,200	1,800
Jan.	2 × 50 =	700		1 × 100 =	700 =	1,400	2,100
Feb.	2 × 50 =	800		1 × 100 =	800 =	1,600	2,400
Mar.	2 × 50 =	900		1 × 100 =	900 =	1,800	2,700
Apr.	2 × 50 =	1,000		1 × 100 =	1,000 =	2,000	3,000
May	2 × 50 =	1,100		1 × 100 =	1,100 =	2,200	3,300
June	2 × 50 =	1,200		1 × 100 =	1,200 =	2,400	3,600
	24 promotions	$7,800		12 promotions		$15,600	$23,400

To staff nurse II = $600/yr = $50/month each; to staff nurse III = $1,200/yr = $100 month each

Promotions

Promotional increases paid to the three levels of staff nurses employed in the ICU (staff nurse I, II, and III) have been documented month by month for several years. Records allow us to make predictions for the future fiscal year, which we will monitor and analyze as the actual promotions take place. Because promotions at various times of the fiscal year have varying impact on the amount of money needed in our budget (i.e., experience differentials) we want to predict their timeliness and cost. Table 9–22 demonstrates how the assumptions may be budgeted. The promotional policy is a $600/year increase to a staff nurse II and a $1200/year increase to a staff nurse III. The Table shows that we have budgeted on the assumption that in any given month two nurses will be promoted to the second level and one nurse to the third level. We can easily monitor variances from the plan and add to historical data as the fiscal year progresses.

The two nurses promoted to staff nurse II in July will require $100 ($50/month × 2) for July. They will require $100 a month for each of the next 11 months.

The two nurses promoted to Staff nurse II in August will require an additional $100 ($50/month × 2) for August. The two nurses promoted in July plus the two promoted in August require $200 to be added to cover the costs of promotional increases paid in August.

In September the two nurses promoted in July and August to staff nurse II will require $200 to be added to the September

TABLE 9–23. PER DIEM BUDGET

	Base Hours	Base ($)	Shift Differential ($)	Total*
July	22 days × 8 hr × 3 = 528 hr × $15.00 =	$ 7,920	22 days × $12.00 = $ 264	$ 8,184
Aug.	21 days × 8 hr × 3 = 504 hr × $15.00 =	7,560	21 days × 12.00 = 252	$ 7,812
Sept.	22 days × 8 hr × 2 = 352 hr × $15.00 =	5,280	22 days × 12.00 = 264	$ 5,544
Oct.	22 days × 8 hr × 2 = 352 hr × $15.00 =	5,280	22 days × 12.00 = 264	$ 5,544
Nov.	21 days × 8 hr × 2 = 336 hr × $15.00 =	5,040	21 days × 12.00 = 252	$ 5,292
Dec.	22 days × 8 hr × 2 = 352 hr × $15.00 =	5,280	22 days × 12.00 = 264	$ 5,544
Jan.	22 days × 8 hr × 2 = 352 hr × $15.75 =	5,544	22 days × 12.60 = 277	$ 5,821
Feb.	21 days × 8 hr × 2 = 336 hr × $15.75 =	5,292	21 days × 12.60 = 265	$ 5,557
Mar.	22 days × 8 hr × 2 = 352 hr × $15.75 =	5,544	22 days × 12.60 = 277	$ 5,821
Apr.	22 days × 8 hr × 2 = 352 hr × $15.75 =	5,544	22 days × 12.60 = 277	$ 5,821
May	21 days × 8 hr × 2 = 336 hr × $15.75 =	5,292	21 days × 12.60 = 265	$ 5,557
June	22 days × 8 hr × 2 = 352 hr × $15.75 =	5,544	22 days × 12.60 = 277	5,821
Total base hr	4,504 Base	$69,120	Shift = $3,198	$72,318
			÷ 52 ÷ 40 =	2.2 FTEs.

*base ($) + shift differential ($)

budget. The cost of the September promotions effected is $100. The total needed for August is thus $300. Continuing the cost impact for the fiscal year, the 24 promotions effected at two per month in our plan, will require $7800 to be added to our budget. The concept is the same for the promotions to staff nurse III. When the monthly costs of both promotion levels are added, the total monthly increase is the result.

Per Diem Nurses

Per diem nurses are employees without a regularly scheduled work week. They do not work a fixed number of hours or days per week. They can be considered as *substitutes* for regularly scheduled nurses who call in sick, or additional staffing when the patient census or acuity is higher than usual, or temporary fill-ins for vacant positions. Per diem staff have no fringe benefits, vacation, sick leave holidays, health insurance, and so on, and usually earn a premium rate in view of this fact. Often the rate is a fixed flat rate, regardless of the experience or skill level of the practitioner. Generally per diem nurses have several years of experience and practice warranting their premium rate of pay.

The ICU records over the past several years show the monthly usage of per diems to be increasing slightly. In view of the predicted vacancy rate, and sick call experience, we plan to budget per diems at three FTEs for July and August and two FTEs for the remaining months.

The salary program for per diem nurses is different than that of staff nurses. A rate of $15.00/hour for an 8-hour shift or $120.00/shift is assumed. A shift differential of 10 percent (or $12.00/shift) for evenings and night shifts is assumed. It is further assumed that *one* of the per diem FTEs throughout the 12 months of the fiscal year will work an evening *or* a night shift; in July and August the remaining two FTEs will work days, and in the other 10 months, the remaining FTE will work days. We will project a salary increase of 5 percent on January 1. Table 9–23 shows the hours (and FTE) budgeted as well as the base and shift differential dollars budgeted each month. Note how the variables change month to month based on our earlier assumptions.

Having calculated budget needs by factors, it now remains to combine these factors in some meaningful ways.

Table 9–24 shows the budgeted factors and the amounts for each according to employee classification. Pictured in this way, one has a short but comprehensive idea of what makes up the salary budget of over $4 million dollars. Expense for each factor and/or each employee group can be easily compared to previous summaries of the same type for previous fiscal years to determine

TABLE 9–24. SALARY FACTOR BUDGET FOR FISCAL YEAR

Factor	Management	Staff Nurses	Aides	Clerks	Total
1. Base salaries	$211,319	$2,770,328	$506,564	$190,502	$3,678,713
2. Shift differential	6,996	216,996	30,702	10,236	264,930
3. Holiday differential		38,519	7,057	2,743	48,319
4. Overtime premium		8,029	2,658	1,182	11,869
5. On-call		36,984			36,984
6. Experience differential	350	4,950			5,300
7. Promotion differential		23,400			23,400
8. Per diems		72,318			72,318
Totals	$218,665	$3,171,524	$546,981	$204,663	$4,141,833
Percent budget	5%	77%	13%	5%	100%

increased costs. As the changes are made from year to year, a budget justification summary should be prepared and maintained for reference (regarding assumptions made) throughout the fiscal year and for historical reference as well. A budget manual should not include the official forms with the numbers, but back-up calculation worksheets as to how the numbers got on the page. The worksheets can be used for noting highlights of changes as they occur during the fiscal year. At the next budget preparation cycle, these notes can be helpful in making better predictions for the next fiscal year.

Once built, the budget has to be "sold" to department heads, administrators, and finance managers. Detailed knowledge regarding what the budget factors are and how they have been calculated can be very helpful in explaining/defending the budget.

Tables 9–25 through 9–28 are monthly salary budgets for each employee classification according to budget factor.

Table 9–29 is a summary of each employee classification's monthly budget. The fiscal year is hence broken down into the 12 monthly budgets. As performance reports are generated each month, the summaries in Table 9–25 through 9–28 can be helpful in comparing the budgeted amounts to the actual expenditures and the budgeted *assumptions* to the actual performance.

Variance analysis of each month's performance, i.e., comparing the budgeted and the actual expenditures and the *reason* for the difference, is important to the budget process. In budget building we have seen how heavily records are relied on, factor by factor, to budget for a particular factor. Our assumptions regarding premium overtime use, on-call use, promotions from staff nurse to staff nurse II and to staff nurse III, per diem use, and even the turnover factor (not budgeting two vacancies) all

TABLE 9–25. MONTHLY SALARY BUDGET BY FACTOR—MANAGEMENT

Factor	Base Salaries	Shift Differential	Experience Differential	Total
July	$ 17,266	$ 583	$ 0	$ 17,849
Aug.	16,481	583	0	17,064
Sept.	17,266	583	25	17,874
Oct.	17,931	583	25	18,539
Nov.	17,116	583	25	17,724
Dec.	17,931	583	25	18,539
Jan.	18,163	583	25	18,771
Feb.	17,338	583	25	17,946
Mar.	18,163	583	50	18,796
Apr.	18,163	583	50	18,796
May	17,338	583	50	17,971
June	18,163	583	50	18,796
Total	$211,319	$6,996	$350	$218,665

rely on records kept on a month by month basis. The variance analysis by factor serves two important purposes; first, it allows you to determine why expenditures are what they are. Anyone can see a number on a report and know *what* the number is, however, variance analysis that compares factor by factor each budget classification, tells you *why* the number is what it is. If one has budgeted two per diem FTEs in December, and the actual expenditures indicated usage of 3.5 FTEs, one can easily document cost and reason for this overexpenditure. If there are four vacancies, instead of the assumed two vacancies, one can easily document this underexpenditure. If no one has been promoted in a particular month, one can estimate the savings for that particular month. All the factors going into the budget need to be analyzed each month to understand the expenditure variance. Knowing what the variance is and why, allows one to take steps to correct any problem in the variance. Significant over expenditure and underexpenditure, actual or projected, can be acted on for corrective measures. This is extremely important for sound fiscal management.

Variance analysis, by its nature, helps in collecting the data necessary to make more accurate budget assumptions. By noting the actual numbers of per diems used, promotions made, and number of vacancies, the record is compiled month by month for use in the next budget preparation period. The better the picture and understanding of the past, the better the picture for the future.

Second, the budget process is cyclical. Everything builds each month, as actual performance reports are produced and the

TABLE 9–26. MONTHLY SALARY BUDGET BY FACTOR—STAFF NURSES

Month	Base Salaries	Shift Differential	Holiday Differential	Overtime	On-call	Experience Differential	Promotion Increase	Per Diem	Total
July	$ 198,993	$ 18,083	$ 2,692	$ 646	$ 2,746	$ 150	$ 300	$ 8,184	$ 231,794
Aug.	207,110	18,083	0	643	2,734	200	600	7,812	237,182
Sept.	239,691	18,083	3,257	674	3,580	300	900	5,544	272,029
Oct.	239,691	18,083	3,257	674	2,864	300	1,200	5,544	271,613
Nov.	228,796	18,083	9,771	674	2,864	325	1,500	5,292	267,305
Dec.	239,691	18,083	3,257	674	3,580	475	1,800	5,544	273,104
Jan.	239,691	18,083	6,514	674	2,864	475	2,100	5,821	276,222
Feb.	228,796	18,083	6,514	674	2,864	475	2,400	5,557	265,363
Mar.	239,691	18,083	0	674	3,580	525	2,700	5,821	271,074
Apr.	239,691	18,083	0	674	2,864	525	3,000	5,821	270,658
May	228,796	18,083	3,257	674	2,864	550	3,300	5,557	263,081
June	239,691	18,083	0	674	3,580	650	3,600	5,821	272,099
Total	$2,770,328	$216,996	$38,519	$8,029	$36,984	$4,950	$23,400	$72,318	$3,171,524
Percent	87.4	6.8	1.2	0.3	1.2	0.1	0.7	2.3	100

TABLE 9-27. MONTHLY SALARY BUDGET BY FACTOR—AIDES

Month	Base Salaries	Shift Differential	Holiday Differential	Overtime	Total
July	$ 41,184	$ 2,496	$ 576	$ 216	$ 44,472
Aug.	39,312	2,496	0	216	42,024
Sept.	43,056	2,496	576	216	46,344
Oct.	41,184	2,496	576	216	44,472
Nov.	39,312	2,496	1,728	216	43,752
Dec.	43,056	2,496	576	216	46,344
Jan.	43,243	2,621	1,210	227	47,301
Feb.	41,278	2,621	1,210	227	45,336
Mar.	45,209	2,621	0	227	48,057
Apr.	43,243	2,621	0	227	46,091
May	41,278	2,621	605	227	44,731
June	45,209	2,621	0	227	48,057
Total	$506,564	$30,702	$7,057	$2,658	$546,981
Percent	92.6	5.6	1.3	0.5	100

data are analyzed and documented. The documented records are then used, over a period of time, to make budget assumptions for the projected fiscal year. Assumptions based on historical data should always be made in view of planned changes as a result of new program impact, i.e., if positions are added as a result of an overtime analysis, then overtime should be reduced in the budget being planned. As budget predictions are made, they should be documented so that they can be modified as the need indicates.

TABLE 9-28. MONTHLY SALARY BUDGET BY FACTOR—CLERKS

Month	Base Salaries	Shift Differential	Holiday Differential	Overtime	Total
July	$ 15,488	$ 832	$ 224	$ 96	$ 16,640
Aug.	14,784	832	0	96	15,712
Sept.	16,192	832	224	96	17,344
Oct.	15,488	832	224	96	16,640
Nov.	14,784	832	672	96	16,384
Dec.	16,192	832	224	96	17,344
Jan.	16,262	874	470	101	17,707
Feb.	15,523	874	470	101	16,968
Mar.	17,002	874	0	101	17,977
Apr.	16,262	874	0	101	17,237
May	15,523	874	235	101	16,733
June	17,002	874	0	101	17,977
Total	$190,502	$10,236	$2,743	$1,182	$204,663
Percent	93.1	5.0	1.3	0.6	100

TABLE 9–29. MONTHLY SALARY BUDGET—ALL EMPLOYEES

Month	Management	Staff Nurses	Aides	Clerks	Total
July	$ 17,849	$ 231,794	$ 44,472	$ 16,640	$ 310,755
Aug.	17,064	237,182	42,024	15,712	311,982
Sept.	17,874	272,029	46,344	17,344	353,591
Oct.	18,539	271,613	44,472	16,640	351,264
Nov.	17,724	267,305	43,752	16,384	345,165
Dec.	18,539	273,104	46,344	17,344	355,331
Jan.	18,771	276,222	47,301	17,707	360,001
Feb.	17,946	265,363	45,336	16,968	345,613
Mar.	18,796	271,074	48,057	17,977	355,904
Apr.	18,796	270,658	46,091	17,237	352,782
May	17,971	263,081	44,731	16,733	342,516
June	18,796	272,099	48,057	17,977	356,929
Total	$218,665	$3,171,524	$546,981	$204,663	$4,141,833

The budget process is not a once a year exercise in completing forms and guessing about numbers. It is a consistent effort at documenting and analyzing performance against assumptions and improving on predictions. Budgeting is an ongoing, monthly task.

In the next chapter, the nonsalary side of the budget is discussed.

CHAPTER **10**

The Operational Budget of the Nursing Organization: Nonsalaries

Robert Smith

Just as there are a wide range of factors to be analyzed before a *salaries* budget can be built, there are also a wide range of factors to be analyzed in the preparation of a *nonsalaries* budget.

A nonsalary, or nonpersonnel, budget includes the daily supplies consumed and minor equipment used on a nursing unit. The difference between capital equipment (over $500) and operating budget equipment purchases has already been identified. Actually, there are many types of nonsalary expense categories other than supplies and equipment, as will be illustrated. Nonsalary or nonpersonnel includes all operating expenses other than salaries. It is also sometimes referred to as other than personnel salaries (OTPS).

The expense categories are numerous. Most organizations publish a manual of expense codes for users' reference. It usually contains hundreds of codes and definitions of expenses for utilities, fringe benefits, depreciation, telephone, insurance, taxes, licenses, and many other items that most operating departments do not include in their normal operating budgets. For the most part, these types of *overhead* expenses are borne by one department and expenses are allocated based on actual costs, to each department according to specific criteria, i.e., utilities based on square footage, fringe benefits based on employee population.

These costs are generally centralized for budgeting and expense reporting so most nursing units need not concern themselves with them. In the ICU example they will not be considered.

Before we begin the ICU nonsalary budget, we should look at some expense items common to a nursing unit, but not necessarily to an ICU.

Administratively, there will be expenses budgeted for which there is no bed base. Administrative nursing costs are *stepped down* or reallocated to the various clinical services proportionally, traditionally by the cost-accounting department within the finance division. Administrative expenses are centralized for control and accountability purposes. Some kinds of administrative costs that would not necessarily be reflected in the ICU budget are:

1. Employee Recruitment. Some organizations may reflect *all* recruitment expenses in the personnel department's cost center. If the nurse recruiter is in the personnel department, this is appropriate. However, there is still a *staffing* function within the nursing department that screens candidates, assigns them to a specific clinical service, keeps turnover records including transfer requests, and so on. Often, the staffing personnel will attend conventions for recruitment purposes (perhaps along with the personnel recruiter), as well as recruit at nursing schools and colleges. Expenses for brochures, travel, and convention fees could be part of the nursing budget. If the nurse recruiter works out of the nursing department, additional expenses for advertising would be included in the nursing cost center as well.

2. Travel and Convention Fee Reimbursement. It is not uncommon for staff nurses to attend clinical seminars or conferences offered outside the organization. Travel and convention fee reimbursement policies vary, but expenses need to be planned whatever the policy may be. Often these expenses are centrally planned in the nursing budget.

3. Housewide Expenses. Nursing units may arrange for certain services that are provided to every clinical unit without a specific plan regarding how much those services will be used by any particular unit, i.e., a prep team, blood drawing team, escort team, and so on.

The nurse manager may have a policy of inviting a guest speaker each year to address staff on current issues or developments in nursing. Consultants may be planned for various studies that may cross clinical lines. These expenses would generally be included in the administration cost center.

Only a few possibilities have been listed for example purposes. Administrative budgets do tend to be different from clinical budgets. Yet, even when comparing clinical budgets we may find some differences. An emergency room may budget expenses for items it later resells to patients, i.e., canes, walkers. A minor renovation may be planned on a particular unit whereas not on others. Service contracts for maintenance on sophisticated monitoring equipment will have impact only in those areas with the equipment. A budget for a particular service may differ dramatically (or only slightly) from one fiscal year to the next depending on what changes or new programs are planned.

In developing a nonsalary budget, we should look at what the factors of analysis and planning are even before we look at individual expense categories to be budgeted.

1. Volume. What is the average usage for particular supply items? Is it a consistent monthly usage or seasonal? Will usage change in the fiscal period for which you are budgeting? What are the leading indicators that assist in predicting volume?
2. Leading indicators. What data need to be available that impact on spending; patient mix, patient census, acuity, number of births; cesarean versus normal deliveries, number of patient isolation, and so forth.
3. Price. What prices, in the fiscal year being planned, will be in effect and at what times/portions of the fiscal year? What data from the purchasing department and individual suppliers do you need to project prices for the time you will budget? What interdepartmental price changes will impact on your budget?
4. Inventory. Planning for the new fiscal year budget should include money to purchase/replace items that may be needed. What minor (noncapital) equipment do we have on hand? How old and in what condition is it? What is the life expectancy of it? Have we spent money to repair it? How frequently and how much? What would a replacement cost? Have technological advances improved on the equipment used and does it need to be upgraded?
5. Technology. What changes in items used are likely? What effect would disposable versus resterilization have? Changes in supply items in recent past will impact on current budget for only part of fiscal year; what would be a full year impact of changes already made, if any?

6. Capital Budget. What purchases were or are planned in the capital request list that may impact on the operating budget in the fiscal year planned? If an equipment item has a 1-year warranty and it was purchased and arrived last month, the warranty will expire sometime in the next fiscal year. Will you need a service contract budgeted? If you are planning to purchase new monitors next year, what will paper cost? If the monitors have a 90-day warranty, how much will a service contract cost?

As we develop the nonsalary budget for the ICU we will be considering the applicable factors and making some assumptions about them. These assumptions need to be documented. As performance reports are generated, we can compare assumptions to the actual expenditures and the variance reason/factor. Significant variances can be corrected only once the reason for the overexpenditure or underexpenditure is known. These monthly variance notes will be helpful in future budget predictions. The more data for historical reference, the more accurate predictions are likely to be. The following illustrations are of material management and other expense categories.

MATERIALS MANAGEMENT

Medical Equipment

A typical expense item would be an intravenous pole on which various infusion pumps would be hung. Portable intravenous poles may cost $125 each but accommodate three pumps. Surgical patients may require four to five pumps necessitating more than one pole for each patient. A new pole accommodating up to eight pumps is now available. Although they cost $300 each, we can justify their purchase as we would need fewer poles. The plan is to replace three of the old type poles (for nonsurgical patients) and buy six of the new ones (Table 10–1a).

There are three refrigerators for nourishment, medications, and specimens. Because they are being opened and used 24 hours a day, 7 days a week, their life expectancy is approximately 3 years. The oldest one is replaced every year. Because it is counter size, its cost is $175 (Table 10–1b).

Three digital bed scales require batteries, which cost $30 each. The batteries last about 1 year so we will need $90. The chair scale battery costs $20 (Table 10–1c).

TABLE 10–1. MEDICAL EQUIPMENT

a.	Intravenous poles 3 @ $125 each	= $ 375		
	6 @ 300 each	= 1,800		
	Subtotal	$2,175		$2,175
b.	Nourishment refrigerator			
	1 @ $175	= $ 175		175
c.	Batteries for bed scale			
	3 @ $30 each	= $ 90		
	Batteries for chair scale			
	1 @ $20	= 20		
	Subtotal	$ 110		110
d.	Covered linen hampers			
	3 @ $100 each	= $ 300		300
e.	Utility carts 2 @ $110 each	= $ 220		220
f.	Blood pressure cuffs 8 @ $110 each	= $ 880		880
g.	Siderail bed bumpers			
	2 pr. @ $80 each	= $ 160		160
h.	Bed cradle 2 @ $30 each	= $ 60		60
i.	Pressure infusers 15 @ $95 each	= $1,425		1,425
j.	Miscellaneous	= 995		995
			Total =	$6,500

The recent accreditation survey cited the unit for not having covers on linen hampers. To be code compliant, we need to replace all three hampers, which cost $100 each (Table 10–1d).

Most of the equipment in the ICU tends to be of a capital expense nature. This is different from many other clinical areas. Table 10–1 e to 10–1 j lists some additional items. The plan includes $995 in miscellaneous items that may need to be replaced. If the money is not spent, the reason will be identified in the variance analysis. The equipment plan based on current projected costs of items at the time we will actually purchase them requires a budget of $6500.

Medical Supplies

Some of the supply items will be furnished/stocked by the general stores department. These items are commonly used on all clinical units, such as bandages, gauze, specimen containers, thermometers, and infusion cassettes. The general stores charges have been increasing an average of 4 percent per year over the last 3 years, but we are projecting, based on our budget guidelines, only a 3 percent increase next fiscal year. However, as we have

TABLE 10–2. MEDICAL SUPPLIES

a. *General stores*

FYX $375,625	405,675	
FYY $394,406	− 375,625	
FYZ $405,675	30,050	÷ 2 yr = 15,025/yr average increase
	30,050	÷ 375,625 = 8% increase in 2 yr
		8% ÷ 2 yr = 4%/yr average increase

405,675 + 4% = + 16,227 = 421,900
Fiscal year current budgeted $421,900

Fiscal year projection	421,900	421,900	421,900
	× 3% inflation	× 1% (projected impact)	
	+ 12,657	+ 4,219 =	+ 16,876
	Subtotal general stores =		$438,776

b. *Intravenous sets*

Fiscal year X	$ 70,000
Fiscal year Y	84,000
Fiscal year Z	95,000
Fiscal year current	$105,000
Fiscal year projection	$105,000
	+ 3,000 operating room increase impact
	$108,000 ÷ 12 = 9,000/mo
	× 6/mo (July–December)
	$54,000

$9,000
×   5% increase effective January
+ 450
$9,450 /mo × 6 mo = 56,700 (Jan.–June)
Subtotal intravenous sets = $110,700

c. *Sutures*

Fiscal year current budget	= $3,300	÷ 12 mo = $275/mo
6-mo year-to-date	= 1,620	÷ 6 mo + $270/mo

Fiscal year projection   3,300
                            + 300 operating room increase impact
                            3,600
                            ×   3% inflation
                            + 108
                            $3,708

Subtotal sutures	=		$ 3,708
Miscellaneous items	$2,016		2,016

Medical Supplies Total			**$555,200**

projected an impact from the increase of operating room cases on the ICU, we will have to adjust our supplies consumed averages accordingly. We will, therefore, increase the general stores portion of the supplies budget (Table 10–2a).

Medical supplies are purchased from outside vendors. Costs have been $70,000, $84,000, and $95,000 over the last 3 years. The current budget is $105,000. We anticipate the current price holding firm until January 1 of the new fiscal year (6 months). The new price will increase by 5 percent. The operating room increase impact will add another $3000. Table 10–2b shows budget calculations.

The current budget for sutures (which we get from central service) is $3300/year. Looking at the monthly expense reports, we see that in the 6 months to date (through December) we spent thus far $1620. This averages to $270/month and when compared to the monthly budgeted amount ($275) we determine we are right on target. We have costed out the operating room increase impact to be $300 for sutures. The guidelines have advised us to use an inflation of 3 percent. The new budget will be $3708 (Table 10–2c).

The total budget for medical supplies includes a variety of miscellaneous items totaling $2016 (after various inflation rates). Our total budget is $555,200.

Pharmaceuticals

The current budget is $30,000 or $2500/month. The 6-month year-to-date expenditures through December are $16,320 or $2720/month. The analysis shows that some of the drugs are costing more than we predicted, whereas the cost of two new drugs were not included in our estimates. We will project an overspent variance this fiscal year of $2640, or 8.8 percent. This is a significant projected variance we do not want to continue so we will want to build a budget for the next fiscal year considering our projected *actual* expenses for the current fiscal year. The current budget of $30,000 looks like it should be $32,640.

The operating room increase impact study advises the use of additional drugs totaling $1800 according to current actual costs.

In budgeting for next year, we have information from the pharmacy purchasing agent that the cost of certain drugs (equal to 10 percent of the current projected expenses for this fiscal year) will increase by 8 percent, whereas all the remaining drugs (equal to 90 percent of our current projected expenses) will in-

TABLE 10–3. PHARMACEUTICALS

Fiscal year current budget = $30,000 ÷ 12 mo = $2,500/mo
6-mo year to date expense =   16,320 ÷ 12 mo =   2,720/mo

Current projected expenses $2,720 × 12 = $32,640
Current budgeted   = 30,000
Projected overexpenditure variance $ 2,640
Projected percentage variance   8.8%

Fiscal year projection $32,640
                              + 1,800   operating room increase impact
                              $34,440

$34,440 $0
×   10%
− 3,444   × 8% = +   276 = $ 3,720
$30,996   × 5% = + 1,550 = $32,546
Grand total pharmaceuticals = $36,266

crease by only 5 percent. Table 10–3 shows calculations for new budget of $36,266.

Reprocessing/Sterilization

Instrument trays and bed pans are resterilized in the central reprocessing department. The charges have been averaging $200/month this year-to-date. Because the budget is $2500, we are on target. The operating room increase impact study advises adding $15/month for reprocessing charges. In addition, we will need to increase costs by 5 percent for inflation effective January, 6 months into the new fiscal year (Table 10–4).

Equipment Repairs

Service contracts for maintenance on 11 cardiac monitors are budgeted at $13,000 for the current fiscal year. The period of the contract coincides with the fiscal year, and will increase by 10 percent when it expires.

There are currently ten cardiac monitors under a warranty contract that will expire on December 31 of the new fiscal year. We will want to add these ten monitors to the already existing service contract, but for only 6 months (January–June) of the fiscal year.

If the contract for the first 11 cardiac monitors is $13,000,

TABLE 10–4. REPROCESSING

Fiscal year current budget	= $2,500 ÷ 12 mo = $208.33/mo
6-month year-to-date expense (Dec.)	= $1,200 ÷ 12 mo = $200.00/mo

Fiscal year projection $2,500
$\underline{+\,180}$ operating room increase impact ($15,412)
$2,680 ÷ 12 mo = 223.33/mo

$233.33 223.33 × 5% = 11.17 − 234.50	
$\underline{\times\quad 6}$ mo	$\underline{\times\quad 6}$ mo
$1,340 (July–Dec.)	$1,407 (Jan.–June)

$1,340
$\underline{+\,1,407}$
Total budget reprocessing = $2,474

and it will increase by 10 percent, the new contract will cost $1300 more, or $14,300. If there are 11 monitors, each will cost ($14,300 ÷ 11) = $1300 for the year or 108.33/month. The second group of ten monitors will also cost $108.33 each, but for only 6 months or $650 each or (× 10) $6500. We will need a service contract for $14,300 + 6500 or $20,800 (Table 10–5a).

In addition, the remaining 12 monitors are of the old type that can be maintained by the clinical engineering department. An analysis of repair incidents and costs results in the decision to budget an additional $5,000 (Table 10–5b).

TABLE 10–5. EQUIPMENT REPAIRS

a. *Service contract*
11 cardiac monitors @ $13,000
$\underline{\times\quad 10\%}$ inflation
$\underline{+\,1,300}$
$14,300 ÷ 11 = $1,300 each/yr
$ 1,300 ÷ 12 mo = $108.33/mo

12 cardiac monitors for 6 mo
$108.33 × 6 = $ 650 each
$\underline{\times\quad 10}$ monitors
$6,500

Subtotal service contract	$20,800

b. *Clinical engineering*

12 cardiac monitors	$ 5,000

c. *Plant and maintenance*

Other minor equipment	$\underline{\$ 1,000}$
Grand total equipment repairs	$26,800

Other minor equipment serviced by the plant and maintenance department should cost about $1000 in repairs (Table
10–5c). The total budget is $26,800.

OTHER EXPENSES

Printing

The nursing staff has developed, along with the patient relations
department, and ICU brochure (pamphlet) given to visitors of
patients in the ICU. It includes special information pertinent only
to ICU patients. The pamphlet is printed by the hospital's print
shop for 20¢ each. We anticipate handing out about 5000 pam-
phlets (0.20 × 5000 = 1000) $1000 will be needed for pamphlets.

TABLE 10–6. OTHER EXPENSES

a. *Printing*			
Visitors pamphlet 5,000 @ 20¢ each	=	$1,000	
Open heart surgery pamphlet	=	2,000	
Total printing	=	$3,000	$3,000
b. *Educational programs*			
Conference X @ 100 × 3 RNs	=	$ 300	
Conference Y @ 50 × 12 RNs	=	$ 600	
Conference Z @ 200 × 1 head nurse	=	$ 200	
Miscellaneous	=	$1,300	
		$2,400	$2,400
c. *Books and periodicals*			
Book X by	=	$42.00	
Y by	=	$29.00	
Z by	=	$36.00	
Journal X	=	$25.00	
Journal Y	=	$40.00	
Physician's Desk Reference	=	$28.00	
		$200.00	$ 200
d. *Office supplies*			
$15 × 12 mo	=	$180.00	
Kardex for staff	=	$150.00	
		$330.00	$ 330
e. *Minor nonmedical equipment*			
1 Chair for head nurse office	=	$220.00	
2-drawer file cabinet	=	100.00	
Magazine rack/lounge	=	$ 40.00	
		360.00	$ 360
Total other expenses			$6,290

The ICU staff have also developed a pamphlet on open heart surgery. It is given preoperatively to patients/family members as a teaching tool. It will cost $2000 for next fiscal year. We will need $3000 for printing expenses (Table 10–6a).

Educational Programs

Staff development programs can be part of an in-service function within the nursing department as well as include attendance at outside seminars and conferences. For example, the ICU staff include a number of nurses in the critical care nurse's association. Participation in programs to improve the quality of care is encouraged.

How do we budget for these programs? There are many seminars and conferences held that must be evaluated regarding content to be presented and value of the program to staff development and improvement of quality of care.

Program evaluation results in a decision to budget $2400 or $500/month for registration fees for attendance at outside conferences. As staff make requests, we will monitor the spending. Requests will be evaluated according to several criteria such as seniority, skill level, program offered, and cost. We may spend full reimbursement if only one person attends; 1/2 reimbursement if two attend; 1/3 reimbursement if three attend. The staffing schedule needs to accommodate release of nurses to attend these programs. Documentation will be required of attendance, and some summary and evaluation of the program offered should be shared with the rest of the nursing unit (Table 10–6b).

TABLE 10–7. NONSALARY BUDGET

Expense Code	Definition	Amount
10	Minor medical equipment	$ 6,500
15	Medical supplies	555,200
20	Pharmaceuticals	36,266
25	Reprocessing	2,747
30	Repairs—equipment	26,800
35	Printing	3,000
40	Educational programs	2,400
45	Books and periodicals	200
50	Office supplies	330
55	Minor nonmedical equipment	360
	Total	$633,803

TABLE 10–8. SAMPLE BUDGET FOR ICU

5-07-01	$ 218,665	Management
02	3,163,724	Professional RNs
03	546,981	Aides
04	204,663	Clerks
Subtotal salary	$4,134,033	
5-07-10	$ 6,500	Minor medical equipment
15	555,200	Medical supplies
20	36,266	Pharmaceuticals
25	2,747	Reprocessing
30	26,800	Repairs
35	3,000	Printing
40	2,400	Educational programs
45	200	Books/periodicals
50	330	Office supplies
55	360	Minor nonmedical equipment
Subtotal nonsalary	633,803	
Total ICU	$4,767,836	

Books and Periodicals

There may be any number of worthwhile reference texts in ICU nursing of value to the staff. Subscriptions to certain journals may also be of value. Listed are three books and two journals desired for the staff. In addition, the Physician's Desk Reference of the current year will be purchased (Table 10–6c).

Office and Instructional Supplies

Expenses for stationery, forms, clips, notebooks, and so on need to be budgeted. The general stores office supply charges are slightly over $14.00/month so far this year. We have been advised to budget a 50 percent increase and determine we will need $15/ month × 12 = $180. We also need to purchase new Kardex records next year and the price quote is about $150 (Table 10–6d).

Minor Nonmedical Equipment

The head nurse's chair in her office is old and shabby. Replacing it will cost $200, plus $20.00 shipping charges. We want to add a two-drawer file cabinet in the supervisor's office and a magazine rack in the staff lounge. The former will cost $100; the latter $40.00 (Table 10–6e). Table 10–7 shows the completed nonsalary budget and Table 10–8 shows the completed ICU budget for both the salaries and nonsalaries categories.

CHAPTER 11

Prospective Payment Systems and Implications for the Management of Nursing Resources

Ruth R. Alward

The decade of the 1980s is one of great changes in health care payment systems in the United States. In an attempt to control the high rate of inflation in health care, federal and state legislators, as well as insurers and other third-party payers, are moving away from retrospective, cost-based reimbursement for each claim and are moving toward paying a predetermined amount per case. In the retrospective payment system, specified and legitimate costs incurred by the health care provider were paid by the patient or a third-party payer based on either a *per diem* rate or on charges calculated after care was delivered. Under a prospective payment system, the provider receives a fixed amount for each case that is considered to be average in cost and duration or in some instances is based on a predetermined per diem rate. Although surplus payment resulting from excess revenue over expenses for that case, patient days, or procedure can generally be retained by the provider, losses must be absorbed. Health care providers are thus encouraged to function more efficiently so that at least costs of care are covered and, at best, they can retain a proportion of the payment as profit or surplus.

After several years of experimental projects in New Jersey and other states, a hospital prospective payment system for general, short-term Medicare inpatients was signed into law in April 1983 (Public Law 98-21, the Social Security Amendments of 1983). The effects of this law on nurse managers and the nursing profession in general are significant.

One of the most immediate effects of the Medicare prospective payment system was a decrease in the average length of stay and thus in occupancy rates in hospitals throughout the country. Rather abruptly, the nursing shortages of the beginning of the decade were turned into nursing staff retrenchment in many areas of the country, although maldistribution of the nurse supply continued to be a problem. Numerous articles on staffing methodologies and reduction techniques began appearing in the nursing administration journals. In 1986, professional nurse shortages again were prevalent throughout much of the country as the supply of nurses failed to meet the demand.

Staffing problems have through the course of nursing history consumed much of the nurse manager's time and energy. The conflict that has always existed between the demands of the health care administrator for high nursing productivity (output as a function of input, or, output : input) and the quest of individual nurses to fulfill both professional and personal goals has escalated with the intensified efforts to contain health care costs.

Understanding the reasons for the change in third-party payer reimbursement will help the nurse manager adjust to what is becoming a major revolution in health care. In this chapter, the development and main features of the current very complex federal prospective payment system are described briefly. Some general advantages and disadvantages of prospective payments systems vis-à-vis the previous cost-based reimbursement systems are outlined. The rest of the chapter is concerned with the implications of prospective payment on the nursing profession and suggests how nurse managers can meet the challenges resulting from the changes in health care financing through modern management concepts of staffing, cost analysis, innovation, and marketing.

Whether or not the most prevasive classification scheme, called diagnosis related groups (DRGs), survives the decade as the basis for prospective payment systems, there will certainly be no return to cost-based reimbursement for health care. If the DRG scheme does not prove effective, the federal government would consider a voucher system through which consumers purchase health care or perhaps allocation of health care dollars on a regional or state basis. Some form of prospective payment scheme will be in effect and the nurse manager will be responding to its impact on nursing practice.

THE MEDICARE PROSPECTIVE PAYMENT SYSTEM

Development of the DRG System

Although the term *health* is not found in the Constitution of the United States, the federal government has been assuming an increasingly more prominent role in providing health care services to its citizens. Whereas former generations assumed personal responsibility to keep healthy, and to care for their sick and frail elderly family members, as taxes have increased the public has come to expect more from the government in return. High on the list of expected benefits has been health care at a reduced or preferably no direct cost to the individual. Now hundreds of health care bills are introduced in each session of Congress. Through the Medicare and Medicaid programs alone, the American taxpayer was paying over two-thirds of all hospital bills by 1980 (Davis, 1983).

After the Medicare program for the elderly and the Medicaid program for the medically indigent were initiated in the mid-1960s, the cost of health care funded by the federal government went from approximately $3 billion in 1960 to $6 billion in 1966 when claims were first paid, and to $51 billion in 1982. Total health care costs in the United States in 1982 were $321 billion or 10.4 percent of the Gross National Product (all goods and services produced), an increase from 6 percent in 1966 (Davis, 1983). Between 1965 and 1982, consumer prices increases 250 percent, whereas health care costs rose 550 percent. The cost-based reimbursement system was criticized for providing financial incentives to keep patients in the hospital longer than was medically necessary and to administer more tests, treatments, and services than were needed. There were no financial incentives for efficiency on the part of hospitals. Instead, the emphasis was on providing health care of the highest quality in the world, regardless of the cost or who was paying the bills.

When it became apparent in 1982 that the solvency of the Medicare trust funds was in jeopardy, Congress passed the Tax Equity and Fiscal Responsibility Act (TEFRA) and asked the Department of Health and Human Services (DHHS) to report on prospective payment for Medicare hospitalization. Following this report, Public Law 98-21 was quickly signed into law in April 1983, and the DRG prospective payment system for hospitalization of Medicare patients was established. It is administered by the Health Care Financing Administration (HCFA). This agency was ably headed by a registered nurse, Carolyne Davis, from 1981 to 1985.

Description of the DRG System

The Medicare prospective payment system is based on a medical classification scheme of DRGs. The DRG classification was developed with federal funding at Yale University during the 1970s as a system for monitoring quality of medical care and utilization review. The classifications were updated and expanded in 1979 to reflect the ninth revision of the International Classification of Diseases (ICD-9). The ICD-9 codings were divided into 23 organ system groups called major diagnostic categories (MDCs). In turn, each MDC was subdivided into 467 DRGs. Three other code numbers (DRGs 468–470) were added for administrative purposes and 471 has now been added for certain bilateral joint procedures. The groupings were based on a study of 1.4 million patients discharged from 332 hospitals in 1979.

Assignment to a specific DRG is made by the GROUPER computer program according to the patient's primary and secondary discharge diagnoses, age, specific complications and/or comorbidity, operative procedures, and type of discharge. Each DRG has a unique decision tree in this program (Fig. 11–1). The determination of DRG is based on information taken from the discharged patient's medical record abstract after certification by the attending physician and sent on the bill to the fiscal intermediary for the Medicare program. Hospitals may also purchase the GROUPER software so that administrators can themselves determine the probable DRG assignment and payment.

In this system the hospital's output or *product* is defined by its case mix of patients assigned to specific DRGs. Patients assigned to the same DRG are supposed to be relatively homogeneous in regard to use of resources during their hospital stays. Because actual costs of care were not known, length of stay was used by the Yale development team to indicate costs when they statistically created the DRGs. Each DRG was also weighted to show the relationship of its costs to the overall average costs of a Medicare patient's hospital stay. Each participating hospital has a case-mix index based on a sample of Medicare patients. This index allows comparison among hospitals in the complexity of case mix. An index of 1 is considered to be average.

For the time being, the federal DRG prospective payment system applies to all inpatient services furnished to Medicare patients by most participating acute-care hospitals. Long-term care facilities, psychiatric, rehabilitation, and children's hospitals and defined units of these types within general hospitals have been excluded. Special payment provisions apply to hospitals that are designated *sole community providers* because they are the

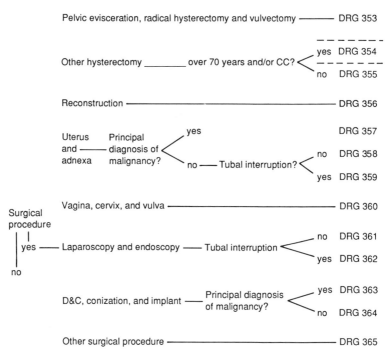

MAJOR DIAGNOSTIC CATEGORY 13

Diseases and disorders of the female reproductive system

Figure 11-1. DRG decision tree: DRG 354 hysterectomy on patient over 70 and/or with complications/comorbidity.

only facility within a large area or are located in an area where access is difficult. Additional payments are also made to hospitals serving a disproportionate share of low-income and Medicare patients. Adjustments and exemptions have been made for major regional referral centers, a few cancer research and treatment facilities, and for hospitals in Alaska and Hawaii. In 1983, the states of New Jersey, Maryland, Massachusetts, and New York were given waivers to continue their own prospective payment systems for limited periods of time and subject to reapplication. When Massachusetts' and New York's waivers expired at the end of 1985, hospitals in those states joined the federal program for Medicare payment.

Inpatient (routine, ancillary, and intensive) service costs other than physician and nurse anesthetist services are included in the DRG rate. Up to October 1986, capital expenses had been reimbursed on a cost basis. Gradually capital payments will be reduced beginning with a .5 percent cut in 1987. Direct teaching costs for medical and nursing education were paid on a reasonable costs basis for the first 2 years of the program, but HCFA imposed a freeze on the third-year payments for direct medical education costs. Future reimbursement for medical education is subject to a hospital-specific limit, but direct-education costs for nursing and allied health personnel continue to be reimbursed on a cost basis. Indirect medical education costs (for interns and residents) are paid to hospitals on a variable cost basis.

Each year, in response to the increasing pressure to curtail health care costs for this growing segment of the population, charges are made in the Medicare prospective payment program, closing loopholes found to be inflationary. Further refinements are expected in the system when the results are available from six projects HCFA funded to study the intensity of care within each DRG. Targeted for further scrutiny, elimination, or prospective payment are for-profit hospitals' return-on-equity payments, physicians' payment, ambulatory surgery, and long-term care. Predictions have been made that by 1990, there will be some form of prospective payment for all types of health care providers and by all types of health insurers.

Implementation

A 3-year period was provided for implementing the Medicare DRG program, beginning with the start of each hospital's fiscal year after October 1, 1983. Each year the payment to the hospital was to be based less on its own previous costs and those of regional hospitals and more on national hospital costs averages. By the fourth year of the program in 1987, each hospital was to be paid according to the national urban or national rural rate. In 1986, the transition period was lengthened to 4 years instead of 3 years.

Payment in addition to the DRG rate is made for atypical cases when either the number of days or the costs of care are excessive. These atypical cases are called outliers. There is a limit to outlier payments made to each hospital and they receive thorough scrutiny before payment.

If a patient is transferred from one hospital to another, the last hospital treating the patient receives the full DRG rate, plus outlier payments if indicated. The transferring hospital receives a per diem rate based on the number of stayed days relative to the average length of stay for that DRG.

Quality Control

Hospitals receiving Medicare payments are required to contract with a peer review organization (PRO) for an ongoing review of their compliance with program objectives for utilization and quality. Each state has its own PRO made up of physicians, or with access to physicians, for review of medical services. All of the individual contracts between HCFA and PROs identify for intensive review specific diagnoses, procedures, and DRGs.

General utilization standards for the PROs to follow are: (1) reduce inpatient admissions for procedures that can safely and effectively be done on an outpatient basis, (2) reduce unnecessary admissions or treatment for specific DRGs, and (3) reduce inpatient admissions or invasive procedures by specific hospitals and practitioners. To prevent unnecessary admissions and inpatient treatment that should be provided in an outpatient setting, preadmission review is mandated for specified procedures and conditions. If a hospital does not comply with this review, it is subject to denial of payments.

Quality objectives of the PROs are to reduce readmissions caused by substandard care during the previous admission, ensure that necessary services are provided, reduce unnecessary surgery, treatment, complications, and deaths. Many variations exist in the specific diagnoses and procedures each PRO has targeted for scrutiny (see Grimaldi and Micheletti, 1985). The PROs are also reviewing all preadmissions within 15 days of discharge, all pacemaker implantations, all cost and day outliers, and a sample of cases to validate diagnoses and the assigned DRG codes. Since the introduction of the DRG program and PRO, hospital occupancy rates have declined to approximately two-thirds of licensed capacity nationwide, whereas ambulatory services have increased significantly.

Advantages and Disadvantages of Prospective Payment

With several years of history now available from New Jersey and an increasing data base from the Medicare DRG program, a few of the advantages of prospective payment are apparent.

1. Hospitals now have explicit financial incentives to provide more efficient patient care, combining economy with effectiveness, as they are responsible for meeting costs that exceed the reimbursement level and can keep in reserve any funds collected above their costs.
2. Hospitals are encouraged to be more prudent buyers of products and services because costs are not automatically passed on to health care consumer.
3. There is increased competition among hospitals and other health care providers for market share. If nurses can show they provide cost-effective health care services that sub-

stitute for more expensive types of care, their share of the market is expected to grow.

4. Hospital revenues are more predictable; therefore, long-range planning can be more predictable. Under the cost-reimbursement system, audits were several years behind and often payment was denied for costs that were incurred years before the audit. (Congressional budget problems have caused some difficulties in planning when new regulations and legislation are passed close to the beginning of a hospital's fiscal year.)

5. The DRG system provides a defined hospital product because discharges (output) are now divided into categories. This has forced hospitals and nursing organizations to find out what it costs to produce each type of service (each DRG).

6. The system helps hospital administrators monitor the effectiveness of various physicians and other health care providers in producing the product (a discharged patient). Practitioners who require unusual amounts of resources in treating a specific DRG or whose practice is unusual when compared to peers are closely scrutinized. A new relationship between the hospital and the attending physician has evolved because of the financial risk to the hospital if costs exceed the DRG payment due to length of stay or use of services. (Physicians may not see this as an advantage.)

7. Ambulatory and preventive health care services are expanding. Hospitals and other providers are opening primary care centers, outpatient surgery facilities, home health agencies, and wellness and other preventive care centers. Opportunities abound for nurse entrepreneurs in many of these outpatient care markets.

The Medicare prospective payments system as it has evolved is not without disadvantages to the health care providers and also to the Medicare patient.

1. Notwithstanding the efforts of the PROs, there is still much concern about the impact of prospective payment on the quality of patient care. Shorter hospital stays, especially for the frail elderly, are resulting in instances of undertreatment and premature discharge of this segment of the population. Patients are being discharged with insufficient rehabilitation and are too often unable to cope with their conditions at home.

2. Hospitals may not be willing to treat patients with diagnoses found to require more resources than are reim-

bursed. There is concern that hospitals are refusing to treat or are transferring (known as dumping in this industry) more indigent patients as a result of curtailment of the Medicare and Medicaid programs.

3. Although the use of nursing resources and the patients' severity of illness within a single DRG may vary significantly, this variation has not been adequately factored into the present prospective rates. Nursing costs in the Medicare DRG system are allocated to each patient according to the length of stay in the hospital and are not related to nursing resources used for the average patient in each DRG. Teaching hospitals are particularly concerned about the availability of only partial reimbursement for outliers who require more care than the average patient. Hospitals treating a disproportionate share of elderly and low-income patients claim that they have been underpaid by the Medicare system.

4. The established prospective rates must be revised frequently to reflect the current state of health care technology or Medicare patients may be increasingly denied these innovations. This involves reweighting the DRGs as hospital practice patterns change.

The de facto health care rationing process has been augmented by adding Medicare patients to the population whose claim to unlimited health care will more frequently be denied. Without clear guidelines for providers and consumers alike, more dissatisfaction and litigation are predicted.

IMPLICATIONS OF PROSPECTIVE PAYMENT

Staffing and DRGs

An early consequence of the DRG programs implemented in New Jersey in 1980, and throughout the country in 1983 and 1984 for most Medicare patients, was an acceleration of the gradual decrease in the average length of stay (LOS) that began in the 1970s. The average LOS for Medicare patients declined from over 15 days in 1975 to less than 8 days in 1985. Although admissions and staffed beds are still declining in some areas of the country, there has recently been a slight increase in LOS as a larger proportion of the less complicated cases are treated in outpatient facilities. The average inpatient is more acutely ill and/or dependent on nursing care. The *easy* patients formerly scattered throughout the nursing assignments are now found convalescing at home. Because patients tend to be sicker when they are admitted and when they are discharged, nursing practice and staffing have been affected.

Nursing managers are using patient classification systems (see Chap. 7) to document increasing needs for nursing care and to justify more nursing hours per patient day. These systems are also used to justify an increased percentage of registered nurses to meet the escalating demands for sophisticated nursing care. The predicted generalized move toward delegation of nursing activities from registered nurses to less educated personnel does not seem to be occurring to any great extent. Some nursing administrators have argued successfully against substitution of ancillary staff for registered nurses in light of sicker patients and the technological advances in health care. With LOS now so important to the financial well-being of the hospital, preventing complications becomes urgent. For the same reason, under the prospective payment system there is greater emphasis on early discharge planning and patient teaching skills of the registered nurse. More of these types of nursing activities must be incorporated into the daily plan of care because of the compressed hospital stay. The result of these changes has been that licensed practical nurses and nursing assistants were subjected to cutbacks and layoffs before the registered nurses in many hospitals.

Registered nurses have not been immune to the effects of the changes in health care financing. Some hospitals have closed and national hospital occupancy rates are at approximately two-thirds of licensed capacity and continuing to drop. Between 1983 and 1985 professional nurses in many areas of the country were terminated and found it difficult to obtain full-time positions. The part-time ranks continued to grow as nursing productivity was increasingly monitored and controlled. But as the number of hospital nurses shrank, job opportunities were increasingly available in home health, ambulatory and long-term care facilities, and in alternative delivery systems such as health maintenance organizations and freestanding emergency and primary care clinics.

In acute-care facilities, greater fluctuation in daily census, closed units, shortages of professional nurses, and reductions in the scheduled number of nursing personnel have intensified staffing challenges for the nurse manager. Prospective payment has emphasized the importance of variable staffing techniques (also called flexible or controlled variable staffing) in managing fiscal resources. Variable staffing means that the number and/or skill mix of nursing personnel on each shift, each day, is adjusted according to the changes in patient census and the projected patient needs for nursing care. The variation in nursing workload is usually calculated based on patient classification systems and the unit manager's professional judgment. Variable staffing must be congruent with the nursing budget, and requires a flexible budgeting approach to be successful (Kirby and Wiczai, 1985). It also requires more skill and effort on the part of the nursing manager.

A core or basic level of staffing is scheduled for the unit based on mean or median census and on historical and projected data that describe the percentage of patients in each category of the PCS (Table 11–1). The core staff is supplemented or reduced according to the predictive workload index of the PCS before each shift begins (see Chap. 7). The more the census or the patient care needs fluctuate on a particular unit, the greater the need for flexible staffing techniques to conserve resources, and the greater the challenge to implement.

Fixed or inflexible staffing describes levels that do not vary according to workload factors. Unless the workload changes little from day to day, fixed staffing plans result in overstaffing and understaffing. Staffing plans are often designed for occupancy levels above the average daily census because the memory is longer for the understaffed days than the overstaffed ones, and there is a desire to be prepared for any eventuality. According to Gillies (1982), a hospital will pay for 1 to 2 extra nursing hours per patient day over PCS requirements and actual nursing hours

TABLE 11–1. CALCULATING OF CORE OR BASIC STAFFING LEVEL

Medical–surgical unit			Total capacity	= 40 beds	
			Average daily census	= 30	
			Average occupancy rate	= $\frac{30}{40}$	= 75%
			(past year)		

Historical PCS data (past year)

	%		ADC	*Daily No. of Patients/Category*	*Standard NHPPD*	*Daily Nursing Hours Required*
Category 1	10%	×	30	3	2	6
Category 2	15%	×	30	4.5	4	18
Category 3	50%	×	30	15	5	75
Category 4	25%	×	30	7.5	7	52.5
						151.5

$$\text{Core staffing (No. shifts/day)} = \frac{\text{Total daily nursing hours}}{\text{Hours/shift}} = \frac{151.5}{7.5} = 20.2 \text{ shifts/day}$$

delivered when variable staffing is not used. The hypothetical cost of this 1 nonproductive hour per patient day (not delivered directly or indirectly to patients) can exceed $3 million annually in a 500-bed hospital with a 70 percent occupancy rate (Table 11–2).

One common approach to understaffing is a registry operated by the nursing organization (also called per diem lists, in-house pools). In 1983 almost 60 percent of hospitals used this technique and the percentage may by now have increased due to prospective payment. There are many advantages of hospital registries over the use of supplementary nurses from proprietary agencies, including organizational control of the nurse. Float pools are another approach to flexible staffing. Premium pay for the cross-trained nurse, willing and able to function in several areas of the hospital, may be cost-effective. Permanent and on-call part-time nurses have come to be necessary to provide adequate coverage when nurses work alternate weekends.

It is more difficult for the nurse manager to correct over-staffing than understaffing. Voluntary or required absence days have been more frequent since the prospective payment reductions. Limits on floatation and required absence in some collective bargaining contracts have reduced the ability of nurse managers to respond to overstaffing.

Nursing Cost Analysis

The Medicare prospective payment system has been a management asset to nurse managers by providing them with information on the use and cost of nursing resources that was difficult if not impossible to obtain before 1983. Cost information is being developed by many nursing organizations related to the consump-

---

TABLE 11–2. ANNUALIZED COST OF 1 NURSING HOUR PER PATIENT DAY IN A 500-BED HOSPITAL AT 70 PERCENT OCCUPANCY RATE/YEAR

500 beds × 70% occupancy rate = 350 average census
    350 patient days × 365 = 127,750 patient days/year

Cost of 1 hour of nursing care = $26.00
    $20 = hourly rate plus overhead for nursing
            administration, secretarial, staff education, etc.
    $ 6 = 30% fringe benefit costs
    $26

$26 × 127,750 patient days/year = $321,500/year

tion of nursing resources for specific DRGs. Most of these studies use PCS data as the basis for assigning nursing costs to DRGs. (For examples for this methodology see Ethridge, 1985; Mitchell, Miller, Welches, and Walker, 1984; Sovie, Tarcinale, Vanputte, and Stunden, 1985; and Shaffer, 1985.) Briefly, these methods use the standard direct and indirect nursing hours allotted to each category of the PCS to establish the average cost of nursing care to a patient in a specific DRG (see Chap. 7). Large standard deviations of the average nursing hours required within each DRG demonstrate the great variation of nursing care needs within the specific DRG (Sovie et al., 1985).

Variable billing for nursing services based on a similar use of the PCS to establish nursing costs per category has been practiced by a limited number of nursing organizations since the early 1970s (Higgerson and Van Slyke, 1982). When nursing costs are known and when nursing charges and revenues are separated from those of room and routine services, nursing's contribution to profitability of the hospital can be analyzed by unit and by DRG. It is the expectation of many nursing administrators that prospective payment will provide the impetus to make this practice universal. Recognizing the nursing organization's contribution to revenue will lead to increase control over its practice and its budget.

Cost analysis by nursing unit, as well as by DRG, becomes increasingly important in the era of prospective payment systems. Only when each nursing unit is a separate responsibility center can the nurse manager have access to the management information required to be fiscally responsible and responsive. Computer systems will increasingly be used to track costs, revenues, budget variances, and the like, by responsibility center and by DRG, or by improved categories of resource consumption that may evolve.

Halloran and Kiley (1984) recommend a computerized nursing information system (NIS) to assist managers in the control and analysis of nursing resources. In their method, nursing diagnoses rather than PCS categories describe the patient. Education, experience, performance evaluation, and wages are variables used to describe the nurse providing care and to calculate the cost of care. The nursing management reports generated by the NIS are used to allocate staffing and to analyze costs. The system was meant to be the nursing complement to the DRS system that Halloran and Kiley describe as a *medical management system* because medical diagnoses are the basis of quantification. They point out that the management of hospital patients relates not only to medical condition but also to needs for nursing care and the social networks.

Innovation—A Necessity

Prospective payment systems present nurse managers at all levels the opportunity to strengthen their positions on health facility management teams or in more entrepreneurial nursing activities by being innovative, flexible, and astute in their use of nursing resources. In this climate of cost containment and competition, they can no longer afford to advocate or condone the way things have always been done but must look for ways to conserve resources by *working smarter*. Clearly, new directions and activities are needed to thrive in this changed health care environment.

Luck and inspiration are not sufficient. Drucker (1985, p. 67) points out that innovation is "a systematic management discipline . . . the effort to create purposeful, focused change in an enterprise's economic or social potential." His list of innovation opportunities includes circumstances that the Medicare prospective payment system has presented to the nursing profession: industry and market changes, incongruities, process needs, unexpected events, demographic changes, changes in preception, and advances in knowledge. New types of information can also lead to "creative leaps of imagination" and innovative practices (Kanter, 1985, p. 1179). Many new types of information, now available to nurse managers, are the direct result of the prospective payment system.

Innovations must be focused on attaining the nurse manager's vision of excellence in practice with fewer resources. Expectations about nursing services must be assessed and revised. This assessment is one aspect of the strategic or long-range plan that nurse managers should develop for the organization. A nursing environmental assessment helps to determine the long-range mission, objectives, and action plans for achievement of objectives. Under prospective payment conditions, this assessment includes:

1. An analysis of patient case mix
2. Changes in patient acuity and dependency
3. Current and projected use of services
4. Competency of nursing personnel
5. Medical staff requirements
6. The community served by the institution
7. Collective bargaining environment
8. Physical plant conditions
9. Reimbursement and regulatory climate

10. Strengths and weaknesses of the existing organization
11. Competitors

All day, off-site brainstorming sessions may be productive for nursing leadership groups analyzing the nursing environment and searching for innovations in practice.

Forced reassessment of common nursing practices and rituals is necessary. These include older rituals such as routine vital signs, charting methods, daily baths, and linen changes. Examples of newer rituals that need assessment are the use of non-standardized nursing care plans, and daily classification of patients without using the data for staffing units. Maid services and nonnursing duties performed by registered nurses must be closely scrutinized as must the nursing care delivery system. Shukla's (1982) research suggested that primary nursing may not be the most cost-beneficial nursing care delivery system on nursing units that lack efficient support systems, especially if the patients do not require highly-skilled care. Group teaching and audio-visual aids have proved their cost-effectiveness in many nursing situations. The sale of consulting services, continuing education, and patient education programs, manuals, forms, checklists, and other tangible products developed by the nursing staff can also be a significant source of revenue and self-esteem for the nursing division and its staff.

Nurse managers should also consider taking back some of the services relinquished to other institutional departments under the cost-reimbursement system. Respiratory therapy is a classic example. The hospital might now find it cost-effective to have nurses perform some of these services, and be willing to give the revenue and extra staff to the nursing division.

Some hospitals are experimenting with rehabilitation, convalescent, and long-term care units managed by nurse practitioners. Nurses can also manage primary and chronic care clinics that are freestanding or hospital-based. Nurse entrepreneurs are establishing new services in health education, fitness, wellness, weight, and substance control, while continuing to operate supplemental staffing and home health agencies (Dayani and Holtmeier, 1984). The list of possibilities is growing and the nursing literature is rich in suggestions of new directions open to innovative nurse managers.

Marketing Nursing Services

One of the types of action plans that flow from the nursing environmental assessment should be a marketing plan for the nursing division, its department, and units. The era of prospective payment and competition for patients has created a new need for nurse managers to develop marketing skills. Their positions and the viability of the organization may depend on these activities. A marketing plan identifies how a group of nurses will seek to identify and respond to the needs, preferences, and perceptions of any other group with whom it exchanges values. It is much more than a promotional or selling effort to increase and satisfy demand for products and services. Marketing goals and strategies may rapidly become obsolete; therefore, the marketing plan has a short range and is revised at least annually.

Rather than using the traditional planning model that begins with organizational goals and objectives and proceeds to strategies, implementation, and evaluation, the Berkowitz and Flexner (1978) market planning model is recommended. It begins with an analysis of the needs and capabilities of nursing personnel vis-à-vis needs, preferences, and perceptions of current and potential consumers of nursing service. The nurse planning group then seeks to broaden the marketing effort by considering not only the nurse, the patient, and the family as markets with which the nursing organization exchanges values, but also other agency personnel, medical staff, volunteers, community, suppliers, governmental regulators, legislators, donors, and professional colleagues outside the organization (Alward, 1983).

The STRAP marketing method described by Sabin (1985) is one that nurse managers will find easy to remember as they incorporate marketing into practice.

S —*Segment* the market into groups of consumers (users) and customers (buyers) with like needs and desires.

T —*Target* one or more segments for a closer look based on the services you can offer and the potential need of the segment(s).

R —*Research* what the targeted segment(s) look for in the service you could provide.

A —*Analyze* the feasibility of providing what these consumers need or desire.

P —*Plan* to meet the needs of the targeted segment by using the four Ps of the marketing mix:
- *Product* or service to be provided and by whom.
- *Place* the services will be given, including accessibility, availability, and design of space.
- *Promotion* of the service to target populations by means of personal persuasion, publicity, and/or advertising.
- *Price* of the service to users, including mental and physical costs as well as dollars.

Just as producing and measuring the quality of a service is often more difficult than making and measuring the quality of a tangible product, marketing a service is in many ways more difficult than marketing a product (Kotler, 1982). Like other services, nursing services are inseparable from the nurse provider. They are consumed as soon as they are produced, are perishable, and cannot be stored. They are also highly variable and depend on the ability and mood of the nurse.

Some of the questions that must be answered to develop an effective marketing plan have been adapted from those suggested by Shaffer (1984).

1. What special skills does this nursing organization (department, unit) bring to the health care arena?
2. Who are the important target groups with which the organization exchanges values?
3. What image of the nursing organization is held by the target groups?
4. What are the primary and secondary services to be offered to each target group and in exchange for what value to the nursing organization?
5. How can the services be improved and more effectively promoted?
6. Which services are profitable and which are not? (Profit is conceptualized here as any gain when compared to the expenditures to produce the service.)
7. Are the services priced appropriately for each market segment and for the financial health of the organization?
8. Who and where is the competition? What action is expected from the competitor?
9. What market data is readily accessible and what must be collected specifically for the marketing effort?
10. What are (or should be) the nursing organization's mission and objectives? Based on the answers to questions 1 through 9, what business is this nursing organization (or should it be) in?

To answer these questions and to systematically monitor the attitudes and the needs of the target groups, a marketing information and research program of varying levels of sophistication is necessary. Existing internal sources of information should be used. These include nursing quality audits and scores, patient and medical staff satisfaction questionnaires, application forms, turnover and absenteeism rates, exit interviews, complaint and grievance records, incident reports, and litigation records. All can provide valuable insight into the needs of patients, nurses and other employees, visitors, and staff physicians, and how well these needs were met. Evaluative comments from professional nurse colleagues, friends, and associates provide indications of the satisfaction of some of the consumers of nursing services. The local newspaper may also be a source of external marketing information. Staff or consultant marketing experts can assist the nurse manager in collecting and analyzing internal and external information and in developing marketing strategies.

The most important aspect of marketing for the nurse manager is developing the "close to the consumer" attitude and the obsession with service that Peters and Waterman (1982) found in excellent companies. Identifying the needs of the individuals and groups the nursing organization seeks to serve in all of its exchange relationships is imperative in the prospective payment climate.

The challenge to the nursing profession to manage creatively its human and fiscal resources has never been greater. Thriving in the era of prospective payment and cost containment in health care demands new skills and innovations in practice. Nursing education and nursing research at all levels of the profession are needed to support the nurse manager's efforts to maximize the use of human and fiscal resources.

REFERENCES AND BIBLIOGRAPHY

Alward, R. R. A marketing approach to nursing administration. Part I. *Journal of Nursing Administration*, 1983, *13*(3):9–12.

Berkowitz, E. N., & Flexner, W. A. The marketing audit: A tool for health service organizations. *Health Care Management Review*, 1978, *3*(4): 51–57.

Davis, C. K. The federal role in changing health care financing. *Nursing Economic$*, 1983, *1*:10–17.

Dayani, E. C., & Holtmeier, P. A. Formula for success: A company of nurse entrepreneurs. *Nursing Economic$*, 1984, *2*:376–381.

Drucker, P. F. The discipline of innovation. *Harvard Business Review*, 1985, *63*(3):67–72.

Ethridge, P. The case for billing by patient acuity. *Nursing Management*, 1985, *16*(8):38–41.

Gillies, D. *Nursing management: A systems approach.* Philadelphia: Saunders, 1982.

Grimaldi, P. L., & Micheletti, J. A. PRO objectives and quality criteria. *Hospitals*, 1985, *59*(3):64–67.

Halloran, E. J., & Kiley, M. Case mix management. *Nursing Management*, 1984, *15*(2):39–45.

Higgerson, N. J., & Van Slyck, A. Variable billing for services: New directions for nursing. *Journal of Nursing Administration*, 1982, *12*(6):20–27.

Kanter, R. M. Innovation—The only hope for times ahead? *Nursing Economic$*, 1985, *3*:178–182.

Kirby, K. K., & Wiczai, L.J. Budgeting for variable staffing. *Nursing Economic$*, 1985, *3*:160–166.

Kotler, P. *Marketing for nonprofit organizations* (2nd ed.). Englewood Cliffs, N.J.: Prentice Hall, 1982.

Mitchell, M., Miller, J., Welches, L., & Walker, D. D. Determining cost of direct nursing care by DRGs. *Nursing Management*, 1984, *15*(4):29–32.

Peters, T. J., & Waterman, R. H., Jr. *In search of excellence*. New York: Harper & Row, Pub., 1982.

Sabin, S. Rehab program's marketing plan was tailored to fit. *Nursing & Healthcare*, 1985, *6*:269–271.

Shaffer, F. Nursing power in the DRG world. *Nursing Management*, 1984, *15*(6):28–30.

Shaffer, F. A. (Ed.). *Costing out nursing: Pricing our product*. New York: National League for Nursing, 1985.

Shukla, R. K. Primary or team nursing? Two conditions determine the choice. *Journal of Nursing Administration*, 1982, *12*(11):12–15.

Sovie, M. D., Tarcinale, M. A., Vanputte, A. W., & Stunden, A. E. Amalgam of nursing acuity, DRGs and costs. *Nursing Management*, 1985, *16*(3):22–42.

APPENDIX A

Leadership Characteristics of Nurse Managers

My interest in studying the leadership characteristics of nurse managers grew out of experience with a management development tool used with graduate students to assess their own leadership characteristics.

The tool, the *Level I Life Styles Inventory* (Human Synergistics, 1979), measures 12 different self-concepts that are based on *Mazlow's hierarchy of human needs* and the *people task* orientation present in the classical leadership theories. The life styles profile is presented in Figure A–1. The 12 styles measured by the Inventory fall into four basic quadrants. In Figure A–1 the upper half of the circle identifies *satisfaction* orientation, whereas the lower half identifies an orientation toward *security*.

The inventory also distinguishes between *people* and *task* orientation as the right and left halves of the circle. The elements of security and satisfaction, coupled with the elements of task and people orientation comprise the four basic styles of the inventory.

- People—satisfaction
- People—security
- Task—satisfaction
- Task—security

The level I of life styles inventory has been widely used in all kinds of organizations and a great deal of descriptive and normative data is available about various occupational groups.

205

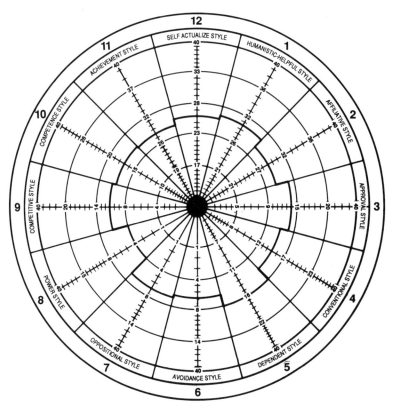

Figure A–1. The level I life styles of a group of potential nurse managers before completion of a graduate program in nursing administration.

A profile of a group of 81 nurses with the level I life styles inventory revealed a profile with dependence as the dominant style. The back-up styles were approval and humanistic-helpful (Human Synergistics, 1979). Although it was not surprising to see nurses described as dependent, I questioned who the 81 nurses were—What was their level of education? What were their positions?

Continued use of the level I life styles inventory as a tool for self-assessment consistently revealed dependence as a primary style. The consistency with which dependence was revealed as a major behavior in would-be nurse managers was striking.

The belief that the completion of a rigorous program of courses in management theory, human resources, and fiscal management, as well as field work in nursing administration, would change the self-concept, and thus the leadership behaviors of these potential nurse managers, led me to formulate the following hypothesis: "Graduate preparation of nurse managers decreases dependency as dominant leadership characteristic."

Dependence is indicative of a need for physical and psychological security as well as concern for neither threatening nor challenging other people. Dependent persons react to stressful situations by doing what they are told, worrying, and/or asking others what they think is right. Dependent managers look to their superiors for direction, forcefully implement goals set by higher management, and rarely act spontaneously. They motivate others by appealing for help in getting what "the boss" needs or wants. (Human Synergistics, 1979)

The changes in the leadership profile of nurse managers after completion of a graduate program in nursing administration closely resemble what has been described as the *ideal profile* with primary and back-up styles in *self-actualization, humanistic-helpful* and *achievement* areas. Individuals with this kind of profile enjoy setting goals, helping others do their best, and are open and spontaneous. They find satisfaction in their lives and in their work (Human Synergistics, 1979).

Table A–1 shows the results of testing with the level 1 life styles inventory in the first semester of a master's program in nursing management, and post-testing of a group of nurse managers 1 year after completion of the graduate program in nursing management. The study revealed a significant difference between the groups in the humanistic style, the dependence style, and the achievement style. There was a significant decrease in dependency $(+(85) = 2.32, p = 0.05)$ for masters-prepared managers.

TABLE A–1. T-TESTS COMPARING PREGRADUATION AND POSTGRADUATION STUDENTS ON 12 SCALES OF THE LIFE STYLES INVENTORY

Variable	Pregraduation Group $n = 67$		Postgraduation Group $n = 20$		
	Mean	SD	Mean	SD	T
Humanistic style	30.9	5.4	33.5	3.9	−2.35*
Affiliative style	30.1	6.0	31.2	4.2	−0.87
Approval style	12.0	5.8	10.1	4.2	1.56
Conventional style	13.4	5.5	11.1	4.6	1.48
Dependent style	15.4	5.8	13.4	2.5	2.32*
Avoidance style	5.3	4.5	3.8	3.1	1.69
Oppositional style	6.7	5.4	5.2	5.0	1.14
Power style	5.3	5.8	4.8	3.6	0.48
Competitive style	10.7	5.9	9.4	5.5	0.92
Competence style	15.6	6.1	17.4	4.8	−1.34
Achievement style	30.5	6.3	33.3	4.1	−2.28*
Self-actualization	28.0	5.7	29.5	4.9	−1.49

*p = 0.05

There was also an increase in the humanistic style and the achievement style of these managers ($+(85 = -1.99$, p $= 0.05$) and (T(85) $= -2.28$, p $= 0.05$), respectively.

A further comparison of the group of master's degree graduates with a group of non-master's degree nurse managers also revealed a significant difference in dependency, *with the masters-prepared nurses having a lower dependency score*. There was also a significant difference in the *conventional style*, again, with the master's degree managers having less conventional responses (dependent style ($+37 = 2.76$, p $= 0.05$) and conventional style ($+37 = 3.06$, p $= 0.05$). The significant changes in scores for dependence, achievement, and humanistic-helpful characteristics give some empirical evidence that graduate education for nurse managers has benefits beyond the cognitive domain. I believe that the pressure for change in nursing organizations will intensify—not diminish—in the coming years and that we will need leadership that is *transformational* rather than *transactional*, to cope with these pressures.

REFERENCES

Lafferty, C. *Level One Life Styles Inventory*. Plymouth, Mich.: Human Synergistics, 1979.

Measuring Motivation Using Expectancy Theory*

Expectancy theory suggests that it is useful to measure the attitudes individuals have to diagnose motivational problems. Such measurement helps the manager to understand why employees are motivated or not, what the strength of motivation is in different parts of the organization, and how effective different rewards are for motivating performance. A short version of a questionnaire used to measure motivation in organizations is included here. Basically, three different questions need to be asked (see Questionnaires 1, 2, and 3).

USING THE QUESTIONNAIRE RESULTS

The results from this questionnaire can be used to calculate a work–motivation score. A score can be calculated for each individual and scores can be combined for groups of individuals. The procedure for obtaining a work–motivation score is as follows:

1. For each of the possible positive outcomes listed in questions 1 and 2, multiply the score for the outcome on ques-

---

*From Nadler and Lawler. In Hackman and Lawler, *Perspectives on Behavior in Organizations*, 1977. Courtesy of McGraw-Hill and reprinted with permission from the authors.

tions 1 (p____O expectancies) by the corresponding score on question 2 (valences of outcomes). Thus, score 1a would be multiplied by score 2a, score 1b by score 2b, etc.

2. All of the 1 times 2 products should be added together to get a total of all expectancies times valences _____.

3. The total should be divided by the number of pairs (in this case, eleven) to get an average expectancy-times-valence score _____.

4. The scores from question 3 (E____P expectancies) should be added together and then divided by three to get an average effort-to-performance expectancy score _____.

5. Multiply the score obtained in step c (the average expectancy times valence) by the score obtained in step D (the average E____P expectancy score) to obtain a total work–motivation score _____.

ADDITIONAL COMMENTS OF THE WORK–MOTIVATION SCORE

A number of important points should be kept in mind when using the questionnaire to get a work–motivation score. First, the questions presented here are just a short version of a larger and more comprehensive questionnaire. For more detail, the articles and publications referred to here and in the text should be consulted. Second, this is a general questionnaire. Because it is hard to anticipate in a general questionnaire what may be valent outcomes in each situation, the individual manager may want to add additional outcomes to questions 1 and 2. Third, it is important to remember that questionnaire results can be influenced by the feelings people have when they fill out the questionnaire. The use of questionnaires as outlined previously assumes a certain level of trust between manager and subordinates. People filling out questionnaires need to know what is going to be done with their answers and usually need to be assured of the confidentiality of their responses. Finally, the research indicates that, in many cases, the score obtained by simply averaging all the responses to questions 1 (the P____O expectancies) will be as useful as the fully calculated work–motivation score. In each situation, the manager should experiment and find out whether the additional information in questions 2 and 3 aid in motivational diagnosis.

QUESTIONNAIRE 1

Question: Here are some things that could happen to people if they do their jobs especially well. How likely is it that each of these things would happen if you performed your job especially well?

	Not at All Likely		Somewhat Likely		Quite Likely		Extremely Likely
a. You will get a bonus or pay increase	(1)	(2)	(3)	(4)	(5)	(6)	(7)
b. You will feel better about yourself as a person	(1)	(2)	(3)	(4)	(5)	(6)	(7)
c. You will have an opportunity to develop your skills and abilities	(1)	(2)	(3)	(4)	(5)	(6)	(7)
d. You will have job security	(1)	(2)	(3)	(4)	(5)	(6)	(7)
e. You will be given chances to learn new things	(1)	(2)	(3)	(4)	(5)	(6)	(7)
f. You will be promoted or get a better job	(1)	(2)	(3)	(4)	(5)	(6)	(7)
g. You will get a feeling that you've accomplished something worthwhile	(1)	(2)	(3)	(4)	(5)	(6)	(7)
h. You will have more freedom on your job	(1)	(2)	(3)	(4)	(5)	(6)	(7)
i. You will be respected by the people you work with	(1)	(2)	(3)	(4)	(5)	(6)	(7)
j. Your supervisor will praise you	(1)	(2)	(3)	(4)	(5)	(6)	(7)
k. The people you work with will be friendly with you	(1)	(2)	(3)	(4)	(5)	(6)	(7)

QUESTIONNAIRE 2

Question: Different people want different things from their work. Here is a list of things a person could have on his or her job. How important is each of the following to you?

	Moderately Important or Less		Quite Important		Extremely Important		
How important is. . . . ?							
a. The amount of pay you get	(1)	(2)	(3)	(4)	(5)	(6)	(7)
b. The chances you have to do something that makes you feel good about yourself as a person	(1)	(2)	(3)	(4)	(5)	(6)	(7)

(Continued)

	Moderately Important or Less		Quite Important			Extremely Important	
c. The opportunity to develop your skills and abilities	(1)	(2)	(3)	(4)	(5)	(6)	(7)
d. The amount of job security you have	(1)	(2)	(3)	(4)	(5)	(6)	(7)
How important is. . . . ?							
e. The chances you have to learn new things	(1)	(2)	(3)	(4)	(5)	(6)	(7)
f. Your chances of getting promoted or a better job	(1)	(2)	(3)	(4)	(5)	(6)	(7)
g. The chances you have to accomplish something worthwhile	(1)	(2)	(3)	(4)	(5)	(6)	(7)
h. The amount of freedom you have on your job	(1)	(2)	(3)	(4)	(5)	(6)	(7)
How important is. . . . ?							
i. The respect you receive from the people you work with	(1)	(2)	(3)	(4)	(5)	(6)	(7)
j. The praise you get from your supervisor	(1)	(2)	(3)	(4)	(5)	(6)	(7)
k. The friendliness of the people you work with	(1)	(2)	(3)	(4)	(5)	(6)	(7)

QUESTIONNAIRE 3

Question: Below you will see a number of pairs of factors that look like this:

Warm weather—sweating   (1)   (2)   (3)   (4)   (5)   (6)   (7)

You are to indicate by checking the appropriate number to the right of each pair how often it is true for you personally that the first factor leads to the second on your job. Remember, for each pair, indicate how often it is true by checking the box under the response that seems most accurate.

	Never		Sometimes		Often		Almost Always
a. Working hard—high productivity	(1)	(2)	(3)	(4)	(5)	(6)	(7)
b. Working hard—doing my job well	(1)	(2)	(3)	(4)	(5)	(6)	(7)
c. Working hard—good job performance	(1)	(2)	(3)	(4)	(5)	(6)	(7)

ANNOTATED BIBLIOGRAPHY

1. See Mitchell, T. R. Expectancy models of job satisfaction, occupational preference and effort: A theoretical, methodological, and empirical

appraisal. *Psychological Bulletin*, 1974, *81*:1053–1077 for reviews of the expectancy theory research. For a more general discussion of expectancy theory and other approaches to motivation see Lawler, E.E. *Motivation in work organizations*, Belmont, Calif.: Brooks/Cole, 1973.

2. See Lawler, E.E., Kuleck, W.J., Rhode, J.G., & Sovenson, J.F. Job choice and post-decision dissonance. *Organizational Behavior and Human Performance*, 1975, *13*:133–145, for further detailed discussions.

3. See Lawler, E.E. *Pay and organizational effectiveness: A psychological view*. New York: McGraw-Hill, 1971, for a detailed discussion of the implications of expectancy theory for pay and reward systems.

4. See Hackman, J.R., Oldham, G.R., Janson, R., & Purdy, K. A new strategy for job enrichment. *California Management Review*, Summer, 1975, p. 57, for a good discussion of job design with an expectancy theory perspective.

5. See Nadler, D.A. *Feedback and organizational development: Using data-based methods*. Reading, Mass.: Addison-Wesley, 1977, for a discussion on the use of questionnaires for understanding and changing organizational behavior.

6. See Lawler, E.E. The individualized organization: Problems and promise. *California Management Review*, 1974, *17*(2): 30–31, for an examination of the whole issue of individualizing organizations.

7. See Lawler, E.E. Job attitudes and employee motivation: Theory, research and practice. *Personnel Psychology*, 1970, *23*:223–237, for a more detailed statement of the model.

8. See Nadler, D.A., Cammann, C., Jenkins, G.D., & Lawler, E.E. (Eds.). *The Michigan organizational assessment package* (Progress Report II). Ann Arbor: Survey Research Center, 1975, for a complete version of the questionnaire and supporting documentation.

INDEX